Table Of Contents

So let's not waste any time & jump right into it!

For beginners, understanding the basics of perfume making is crucial. We will discuss the various techniques and ingredients involved in creating fragrances from scratch. Whether you are interested in making natural fragrances or experimenting with different scent combinations, we have got you covered. Our step-by-step guide will take you through the entire process, from selecting essential oils to blending and bottling your creations.

Aromatherapy fragrance blending is gaining popularity, as people discover the therapeutic benefits of scents. We will delve into the art of creating signature scents for relaxation, stress relief, or even boosting productivity. Learn about the best essential oils for aromatherapy and how to balance the different notes to achieve the desired effect.

Vintage perfume replication is another niche within the perfume-making world. We will explore the techniques used to recreate classic scents from the past, allowing you to experience the nostalgia and elegance of bygone eras. Discover the secrets behind iconic fragrances and learn how to replicate them with precision.

Fragrance layering techniques offer an exciting way to customize your scent. We will provide tips on how to combine different perfumes and essential oils to create unique and complex fragrance profiles. Unleash your creativity and experiment with layering to find your perfect signature scent.

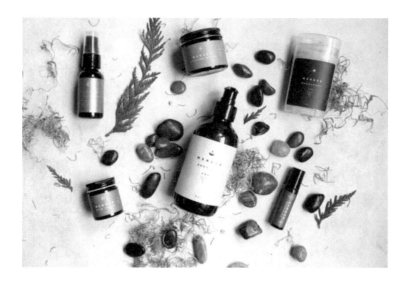

Solid perfume making is a popular DIY project, as it offers a convenient and portable way to enjoy your favorite fragrances. Learn how to create solid perfume balms using natural ingredients and essential oils. We will guide you through the process, from selecting the right base to molding and packaging your solid perfumes.

Customized fragrance oils are in high demand in the e-commerce industry. Discover the secrets of fragrance formulation and learn how to create your own signature fragrance oils for use in candles, bath and body products, and more. We will cover the different techniques and ingredients involved in creating unique and marketable fragrance oils.

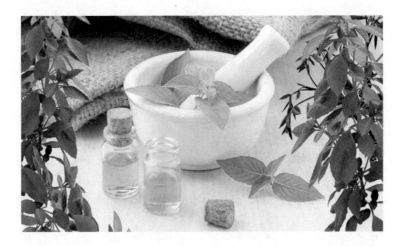

Whether you are a fragrance enthusiast, DIY lover, or an e-commerce entrepreneur, the art and science of perfumery offers endless possibilities. Unlock your creativity, dive into the world of fragrance making, and let your senses guide you on a captivating olfactory journey.

Benefits of Making Your Own Perfumes

If you are a fragrance lover or a DIY enthusiast, making your own perfumes can be a highly rewarding and fulfilling hobby. Not only does it give you the opportunity to create unique scents that suit your personal taste, but it also offers numerous benefits that can enhance your overall fragrance experience. Whether you are interested in creating signature scents, replicating vintage perfumes, or exploring fragrance blending techniques, perfume making for beginners is an exciting journey worth embarking upon.

One of the major advantages of making your own perfumes is the ability to customize your fragrance. Unlike store-bought perfumes that are mass-produced and can be found on countless

others, DIY perfumes allow you to express your individuality and create a scent that is truly unique to you. With a wide range of essential oils, fragrance oils, and other aromatic ingredients at your disposal, you have complete control over the notes, intensity, and longevity of your fragrance. This personal touch can be immensely satisfying and can also make for a great conversation starter when someone compliments your bespoke scent.

Additionally, making your own perfumes can also be a cost-effective alternative to purchasing expensive designer fragrances. By sourcing high-quality ingredients and investing in the right tools, you can create multiple bottles of perfume at a fraction of the cost of a single designer perfume. This not only saves you money in the long run but also gives you the freedom to experiment and explore different scents without breaking the bank.

Furthermore, if you are a DIY entrepreneur or have an e-commerce business, perfume making can be a lucrative venture. With the growing demand for natural and customized fragrances, there is a market for handmade perfumes and fragrance products. By honing your skills and developing your own line of perfumes, you can tap into this market and potentially turn your hobby into a profitable business.

Chapter I: Introduction to Perfume Making

The Art and Science of Perfumery

Perfumery is a delicate blend of art and science, where creativity meets chemistry to create beautiful and unique fragrances. In this subchapter, we will explore the fascinating world of perfume making, offering insights and tips for fragrance lovers, DIY enthusiasts, and those in the e-commerce industry.

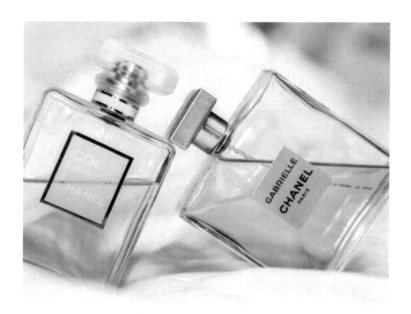

Another benefit of perfume making is the opportunity to explore and experiment with different fragrance combinations. Whether you are interested in creating natural fragrances using essential oils or blending synthetic fragrance oils to replicate a particular scent, the possibilities are endless. You can mix and match various notes, such as floral, woody, citrus, or spicy, to create a fragrance that suits your mood, season, or occasion. This creative process can be both educational and therapeutic, allowing you to deepen your understanding of fragrance families, accords, and the art of perfumery.

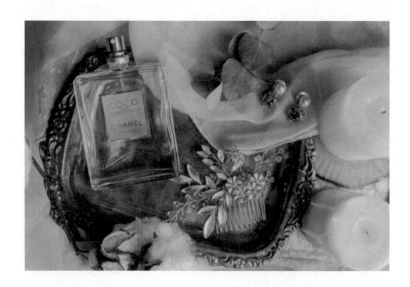

In conclusion, making your own perfumes offers a multitude of benefits for fragrance lovers, DIY enthusiasts, and those interested in the world of perfumery. From the ability to create unique scents that reflect your personality to the opportunity to explore different fragrance combinations and potentially turn your passion into a business, perfume making is a rewarding and fulfilling endeavor. So, if you have a love for fragrances and a desire to unleash your creativity, why not embark on the journey of perfume making for beginners? The possibilities are endless, and the results are sure to be intoxicating.

Essential Tools and Ingredients for Perfume Making

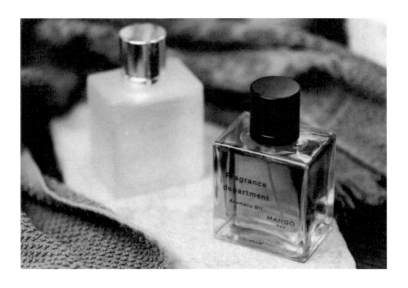

Perfume making is an art that requires the right tools and ingredients to create captivating scents. Whether you are a fragrance lover, DIY enthusiast, or an e-commerce entrepreneur looking to start your own line of perfumes, having the essential tools and ingredients is crucial. In this subchapter, we will explore the must-have items that every perfume maker should have in their arsenal. 1. Essential Oils: The heart and soul of any perfume are the essential oils. These concentrated plant extracts provide the fragrance notes that make a perfume unique. From floral and citrus to woody and spicy, there are endless options to choose from. Some popular essential oils include lavender, rose, bergamot, sandalwood, and vanilla. 2. Carrier Oils: Carrier oils are used to dilute the essential oils and help them blend together. They also provide moisturizing properties to the perfume.

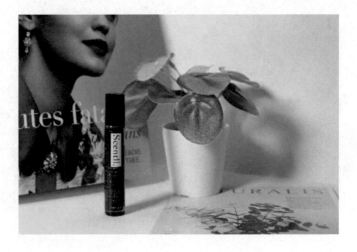

Common carrier oils include jojoba oil, sweet almond oil, and grapeseed oil. 3. Perfumer's Alcohol: Perfumer's alcohol is a specialized type of alcohol that is used as a base for perfumes. It helps to dissolve the essential oils and carrier oils, allowing them to blend seamlessly. It also evaporates quickly, leaving behind the fragrance.

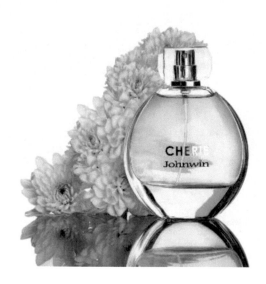

4. Perfume Bottles: The presentation of a perfume is just as important as the scent itself. Investing in high-quality perfume bottles will give your creations a professional and luxurious touch. Look for bottles that are made of glass and have a tight-fitting cap to preserve the fragrance. 5. Pipettes and Droppers: These tools are essential for measuring and transferring small amounts of essential oils and carrier oils. They allow for precise measurements, ensuring that your perfume blends are well-balanced. 6. Mixing Tools: To blend your perfume ingredients effectively, you will need mixing tools like glass stirring rods or disposable pipettes. These tools help in combining the oils thoroughly without causing any contamination. 7.

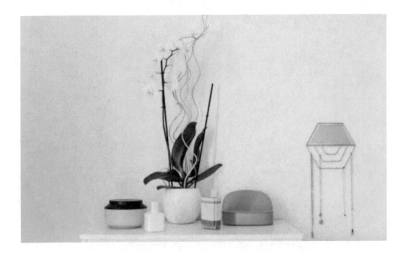

Labels and Packaging: Once your perfume is ready, labeling and packaging are essential for branding and marketing purposes. Invest in high-quality labels that can withstand exposure to perfume oils.

Consider using attractive packaging materials like boxes or pouches to enhance the overall presentation.

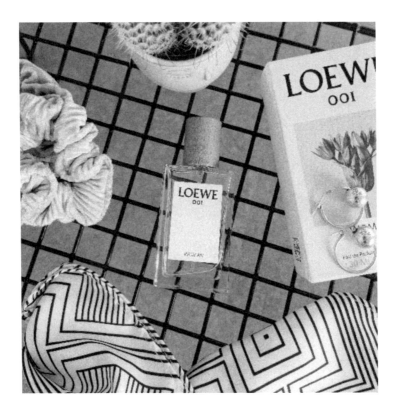

Remember, perfume making is an art that requires experimentation and creativity. Having the right tools and ingredients is just the first step. With practice and a passion for fragrance, you can create unique and exquisite scents that will captivate the senses of your customers. So, gather your essential tools and ingredients, and unleash your creativity in the world of perfume making.

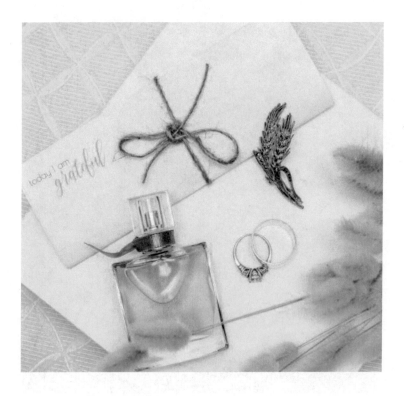

Chapter 2: Getting Started with Fragrance Blending

Understanding Fragrance Notes and Accords

When it comes to the world of perfumery, understanding fragrance notes and accords is essential for creating unique and captivating scents. Whether you are a fragrance lover, DIY enthusiast, or e- commerce entrepreneur, learning about fragrance notes and accords will give you the knowledge and tools to create your own signature scents, explore the art of vintage perfume replication, and even formulate fragrances for bath and body products.

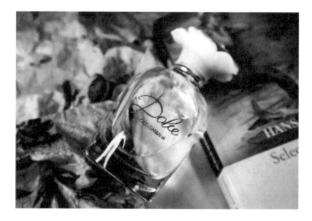

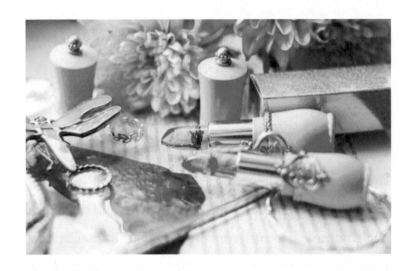

Fragrance notes are the individual components that make up a perfume. They can be categorized into three main categories: top notes, middle notes, and base notes. Top notes are the first scents you detect when you smell a fragrance, often light and refreshing. They provide the initial impression and typically last for about 15 minutes to an hour. Middle notes, also known as heart notes, emerge after the top notes fade. They form the body of the fragrance and can last for several hours. Base notes are the final and longest-lasting scents in a fragrance. They provide depth and stability to the overall composition and can linger on the skin for hours or even days.

Creating fragrance accords involves blending different fragrance notes to achieve a harmonious and balanced scent. Accords can be as simple as a combination of two or three notes, or they can be complex, involving multiple notes from different fragrance families. By understanding the characteristics of each note and how they interact with one another, you can create accords that are unique and captivating.

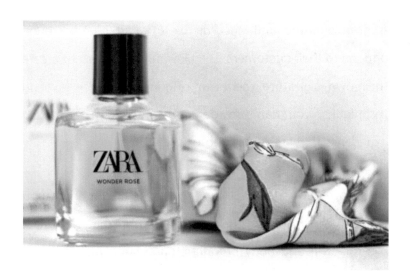

For DIY enthusiasts, learning about fragrance notes and accords opens up a world of possibilities. You can experiment with different combinations to create personalized scents for yourself or as gifts for others. Additionally, understanding fragrance notes and accords allows you to replicate vintage perfumes, capturing the essence of past eras and styles.

E-commerce entrepreneurs can benefit from understanding fragrance notes and accords by offering customization options to their customers. By allowing customers to create their own signature scents or offering fragrance layering techniques, you can provide a unique and personalized experience that sets your brand apart.

No matter your niche, whether it's creating natural fragrances, scented candle making, or formulating fragrance oils for bath and body products, understanding fragrance notes and accords is a fundamental skill that will enhance your creativity and expertise in the world of perfumery. So, dive in, explore, and let your imagination run wild as you unlock the secrets of fragrance notes and accords.

Types of Perfume Concentrations

When it comes to perfumes, there are various concentrations available in the market. These concentrations determine the strength and longevity of the fragrance. As a fragrance lover, DIY enthusiast, or someone interested in e-commerce, understanding the different types of perfume concentrations is essential. In this subchapter, we will explore the various perfume concentrations, their characteristics, and how they can be used in different fragrance-related ventures. 1. Eau de Cologne: Eau de Cologne has the lowest concentration of fragrance oils, usually ranging from 2% to 5%. It is known for its refreshing and invigorating properties, making it ideal for daily use. Eau de Cologne is commonly found in aftershaves and body splashes. 2.

Eau de Toilette: Eau de Toilette has a slightly higher concentration of fragrance oils, typically ranging from 5% to 15%.

It offers a moderate strength and longevity, making it a popular choice for everyday wear. Eau de Toilette is commonly used in perfumes and colognes. 3. Eau de Parfum: Eau de Parfum contains a higher concentration of fragrance oils, usually ranging from 15% to 20%. It provides a long-lasting scent and is suitable for evening wear or special occasions. Eau de Parfum is often found in luxury perfumes. 4. Parfum or Extrait de Parfum: Parfum has the highest concentration of fragrance oils, typically ranging from 20% to 30%. It offers an intense and long-lasting scent, making it highly coveted by fragrance enthusiasts. Parfum is usually sold in smaller bottles and is perfect for creating signature scents or unique fragrance blends.

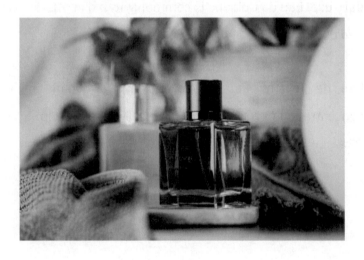

It is important to note that the concentration of fragrance oils affects not only the strength and longevity of the scent but also the price of the perfume. Higher concentrations tend to be more expensive due to the higher quality and quantity of fragrance oils used.

Understanding the different types of perfume concentrations is crucial for DIY projects such as making natural fragrances, creating signature scents, replicating vintage perfumes, or formulating customized fragrance oils. It also plays a role in other fragrance-related ventures like scented candle making or fragrance formulation for bath and body products.

By having knowledge of perfume concentrations, fragrance lovers, DIY enthusiasts, and e- commerce professionals can make informed decisions when purchasing or creating fragrances. Whether you prefer a light and refreshing scent or a bold and long-lasting one, understanding the various perfume concentrations will help you find or create the perfect fragrance for any occasion.

Basic Principles of Fragrance Blending

In the vast world of perfumery, fragrance blending is an art form that allows you to create unique scents that reflect your personal style and preferences. Whether you are a fragrance lover, DIY enthusiast, or involved in the e-commerce industry, understanding the basic principles of fragrance blending is essential to create captivating perfumes, scented candles, and bath and body products. This subchapter will introduce you to the fundamental principles that will serve as a solid foundation for your journey into the world of fragrance creation. 1. Understanding Fragrance Notes: Fragrances are composed of three main notes – top, middle, and base notes. Top notes are the initial impression, middle notes provide the heart of the fragrance,

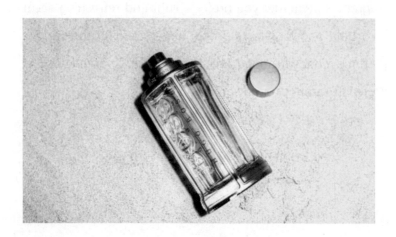

and base notes are the long-lasting foundation. Learning to balance these notes is crucial in creating a well-rounded fragrance. 2. Scent Families: Familiarizing yourself with different scent families, such as floral, citrus, woody, herbal, and oriental, will help you in selecting complementary fragrances for blending. Each family has its unique characteristics and can be combined to create complex and intriguing scents. 3. The Art of Layering: Layering is a technique where multiple fragrances are combined to create a harmonious and multidimensional scent. This technique allows you to customize and experiment with different combinations, enhancing the complexity of your fragrance. 4. Understanding Fragrance Strength: Fragrance strength refers to the concentration of fragrance oils or essential oils used in a blend.

It is important to understand the appropriate strength for different products, whether it's a solid perfume, scented candle, or bath and body product. This knowledge will ensure that your creations have the desired intensity and longevity.

5. Creating a Signature Scent: Developing a signature scent requires experimentation and creativity. By combining different fragrances, you can create a unique and personal scent that reflects your individuality. This principle is especially relevant for individuals interested in creating customized fragrance oils and vintage perfume replication.

6. Natural and Synthetic Fragrances: Familiarize yourself with both natural and synthetic fragrance materials. Natural fragrances are derived from botanical sources, while synthetic fragrances are created in a lab.

Understanding the properties and characteristics of these materials will help you make informed decisions when blending fragrances.

By mastering these basic principles of fragrance blending, you will be able to create captivating and personalized scents that cater to your specific preferences. Whether you are interested in making fragrances for personal use or for commercial purposes, these principles will serve as your guide in the exciting world of perfumery. So, roll up your sleeves, gather your favorite scents, and let your creativity soar as you embark on this fragrant journey of perfume making.

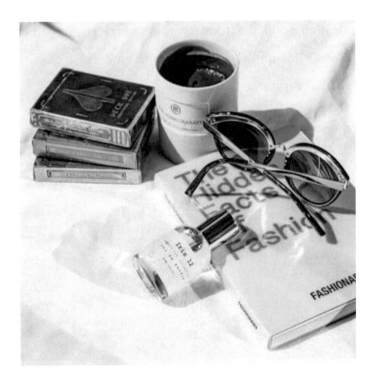

Introduction to Natural Fragrances

Welcome to the enchanting world of natural fragrances! In this subchapter, we will delve into the art of creating exquisite scents using natural ingredients. Whether you are a fragrance lover, a DIY enthusiast, or an e-commerce entrepreneur, this guide is tailored to meet your needs and ignite your passion for perfume making.

Perfume Making for Beginners: A Step-by-Step Guide is your gateway to exploring the fascinating realm of fragrance creation. In this chapter, we will introduce you to the captivating world of natural fragrances and provide you with the knowledge and skills necessary to embark on your own scent- making journey.

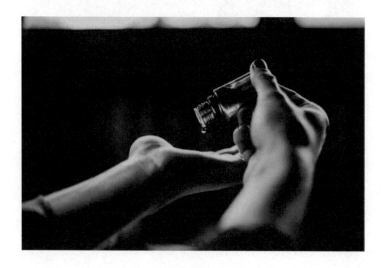

Are you curious about how to make fragrances from scratch? Look no further! We will walk you through the entire process, from understanding the different fragrance notes to blending them harmoniously to achieve a captivating scent. With our step-by-step approach, you will gain the confidence to experiment and create your own unique fragrances.

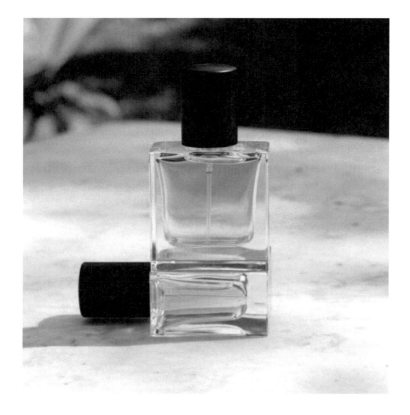

For those interested in DIY natural fragrances, this subchapter will be your ultimate resource. We will explore the wide range of natural ingredients available, including essential oils, absolutes, and botanical extracts. By understanding the properties and characteristics of these ingredients, you will be able to craft fragrances that are not only beautiful but also beneficial for your well-being.

Aromatherapy fragrance blending is another niche we will explore in this subchapter. Discover how to combine essential oils to create scents that promote relaxation, stress relief, or invigoration. Unleash the power of aromatherapy through your own custom blends.

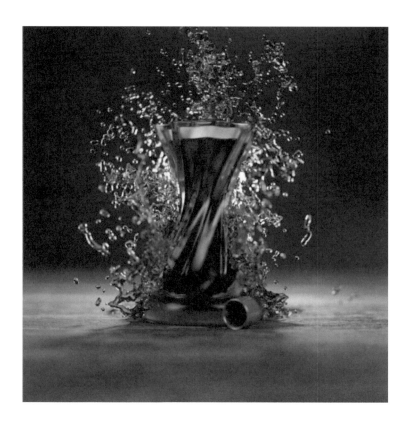

If you have ever dreamed of creating your signature scent, this guide is your key to unlocking that dream. We will guide you through the process of capturing your personality and style in a fragrance, ensuring that you leave a lasting impression wherever you go.

For those intrigued by vintage perfume replication, we have you covered. Learn the techniques and secrets used by master perfumers to recreate timeless classics. Unleash your creativity by putting a modern twist on these beloved fragrances.

Fragrance layering techniques, solid perfume making, customized fragrance oils, scented candle making, and fragrance formulation for bath and body products are some of the exciting topics we will explore in this chapter. Each topic will equip you with the knowledge and skills to expand your fragrance-making repertoire and explore new avenues of creativity.

So, whether you are a fragrance enthusiast, a DIY aficionado, or an e-commerce entrepreneur, join us in this fragrant adventure as we unlock the secrets of natural fragrance creation. Let the art of perfume making ignite your senses and inspire you to create beauty in every scent.

Benefits of Using Natural Ingredients

When it comes to perfume making, there is nothing quite like using natural ingredients. Not only do they offer a range of beautiful scents, but they also bring numerous benefits to your fragrance creations. In this subchapter, we will explore the advantages of using natural ingredients in perfume making.

First and foremost, natural ingredients provide a more authentic and unique scent. Unlike synthetic fragrances, which often smell artificial and generic, natural ingredients offer a rich and complex aroma that is difficult to replicate. This is particularly important for fragrance lovers who appreciate the beauty and intricacy of scents.

Furthermore, using natural ingredients allows you to create DIY natural fragrances. If you are someone who enjoys making your own perfumes, natural ingredients offer endless possibilities for customization. You can experiment with different combinations of essential oils, absolutes, and extracts to create your signature scents that reflect your personal style and preferences.

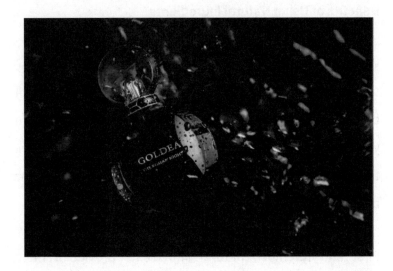

In addition to their olfactory benefits, natural ingredients also have therapeutic properties. Many essential oils used in perfumery have been known for their aromatherapy benefits, such as calming the mind, boosting mood, and promoting relaxation. By incorporating these natural ingredients into your perfumes, you can create fragrances that not only smell great but also have a positive impact on your overall well-being.

Moreover, natural ingredients are ideal for those interested in vintage perfume replication. If you are passionate about recreating historical fragrances, using natural ingredients is essential. Many classic perfumes were formulated using natural materials, and replicating their scents requires the use of authentic ingredients.

Natural ingredients also excel in fragrance layering techniques. Layering scents is a popular practice among fragrance enthusiasts, as it allows them to create unique and personalized combinations. Natural ingredients, with their distinct and complementary aromas, provide the perfect building blocks for layering fragrances, resulting in a harmonious and multi-dimensional scent experience.

Lastly, natural ingredients are not limited to perfumes alone. They can be used in various other fragrance-related products, such as solid perfumes, customized fragrance oils, scented candles, and bath and body products. By incorporating natural ingredients into these products, you can ensure they are free from harmful chemicals and offer a more natural and luxurious experience.

In conclusion, the benefits of using natural ingredients in perfume making are undeniable. From their authentic scents and therapeutic properties to their versatility in various fragrance products, natural ingredients are a must-have for anyone passionate about creating beautiful and unique fragrances. So, embrace the power of nature and let your creativity flourish in the world of perfume making.

Essential Oils and Extracts for Natural Perfumes

When it comes to creating your own signature scent, essential oils and extracts play a crucial role. These natural substances are the building blocks of fragrance, and understanding their properties can help you craft unique and personalized perfumes. In this subchapter, we will explore the world of essential oils and extracts, and how they can be used in perfume making.

Chapter 4: Perfume Making Techniques for Beginners

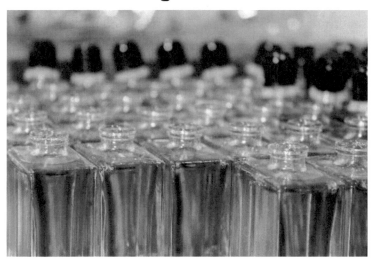

Essential oils are highly concentrated plant extracts obtained through various methods such as distillation or cold-pressing. They are known for their potent aromas and therapeutic benefits. From floral scents like rose and lavender to citrusy notes like bergamot and lemon, essential oils offer a wide range of fragrances to choose from. These oils can be used alone or blended together to create complex and captivating perfumes.

When selecting essential oils for perfume making, it's important to consider their top, middle, and base notes. Top notes are the first scents you smell when applying a perfume, and they tend to be light and refreshing. Middle notes provide the heart of the fragrance, while base notes are long-lasting and give depth to the scent. By combining oils from each category, you can achieve a well- balanced and harmonious perfume.

In addition to essential oils, extracts from various natural sources can also be used in perfume making. For example, vanilla extract adds a warm and sweet note, while benzoin extract provides a rich and balsamic aroma. These extracts can be used in combination with essential oils to add complexity and depth to your perfumes.

Creating your own natural fragrances allows you to customize scents according to your preferences. You can experiment with different combinations of essential oils and extracts, adjusting the proportions to achieve the desired scent. Whether you're aiming for a fresh and invigorating fragrance or a sensual and exotic one, the possibilities are endless.

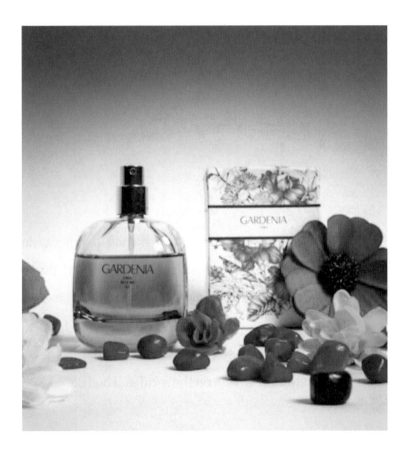

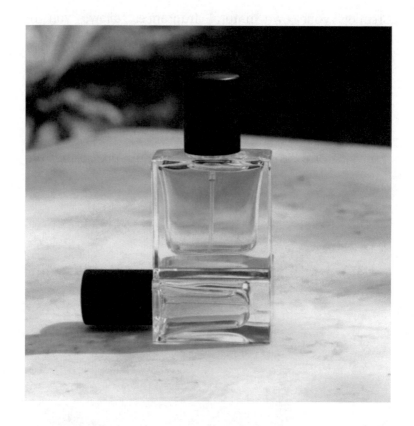

Furthermore, natural perfumes have gained popularity in recent years due to their potential health benefits. Unlike synthetic fragrances, which may contain harmful chemicals, natural perfumes are free from toxins. They can also be used for aromatherapy purposes, as certain essential oils have calming or energizing effects on the mind and body.

Whether you're a fragrance lover, a DIY enthusiast, or an e-commerce entrepreneur, exploring the world of essential oils and extracts for natural perfumes opens up a world of creativity and endless possibilities. From creating your own signature scent to crafting unique fragrances for bath and body products or scented candles, understanding the characteristics and uses of essential oils and extracts is essential for any budding perfume maker. So dive into the world of natural fragrances and let your creativity flourish!

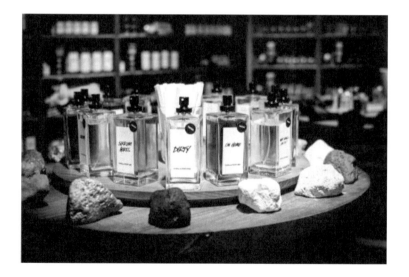

Building a Fragrance Pyramid

In the world of perfumery, creating a fragrance that is both captivating and long-lasting is an art form. One of the key techniques used by perfumers is the creation of a fragrance pyramid. This

subchapter will guide fragrance lovers, DIY enthusiasts, and e-commerce entrepreneurs through the process of building a fragrance pyramid, step by step.

The fragrance pyramid is a visual representation of the different scent notes that make up a perfume. It consists of three layers: top notes, middle notes, and base notes. Each layer contributes to the overall character and longevity of the fragrance.

First, let's explore the top notes. These are the initial scents that you smell when you apply a perfume. They are light, fresh, and evaporate quickly. Common top notes include citrus fruits, herbs, and floral essences. When building your fragrance pyramid, it's important to choose top notes that create an enticing first impression and set the tone for the rest of the scent experience.

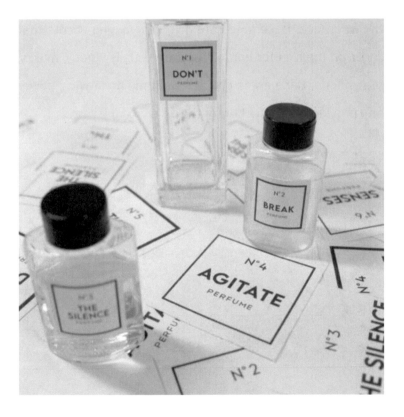

Next, we move on to the middle notes, also known as heart notes. These scents emerge once the top notes have evaporated. Middle notes provide the main body of the fragrance and are often floral, fruity, or spicy. They add complexity and depth to the perfume, creating a captivating and harmonious blend.

Finally, we reach the base notes, which are the foundation of the fragrance. Base notes are rich, long-lasting scents that linger on the skin for hours. They are usually woody, musky, or resinous. Base notes give the perfume its staying power and provide a solid anchor for the other scent layers.

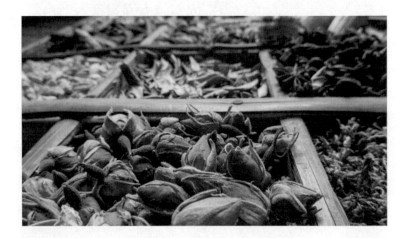

To create your own fragrance pyramid, start by selecting a combination of top, middle, and base notes that complement each other. Experiment with different essential oils, absolutes, and fragrance oils to find the perfect balance. Consider the mood and purpose of your fragrance – whether it's for everyday wear, special occasions, or aromatherapy.

Remember that the fragrance pyramid is just a guide, and you have the creative freedom to customize it according to your personal preferences. Feel free to layer scents, blend different notes, and experiment with unconventional combinations. The beauty of perfume making is that it allows you to create unique and signature scents that reflect your individuality.

By mastering the art of building a fragrance pyramid, you can unlock endless possibilities in the world of perfume making. Whether you're interested in DIY natural fragrances, vintage perfume replication, or customized fragrance oils for e-commerce, understanding the structure of a fragrance pyramid is essential. So, grab your essential oils and embark on a fragrant journey of creativity and self-expression.

Creating Balance and Harmony in Perfume Formulas

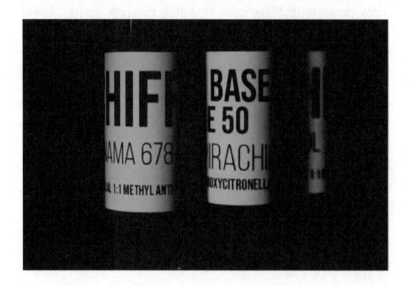

When it comes to perfume making, creating a balanced and harmonious fragrance formula is essential. The art of blending various scent notes to achieve a well-rounded and pleasing aroma is what sets apart a mediocre perfume from a truly exceptional one. In this subchapter, we will explore the key principles and techniques to help you achieve balance and harmony in your perfume formulas.

One of the first steps in creating a balanced perfume is understanding the fragrance pyramid. A fragrance pyramid consists of three layers: top notes, middle notes, and base notes. Each layer plays a crucial role in the overall scent profile and longevity of the perfume. By carefully selecting and combining notes from each layer, you can create a fragrance that evolves beautifully over time.

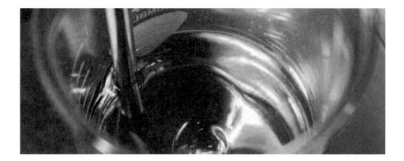

Another important aspect of creating balance and harmony is understanding the concept of scent families. Scent families are groups of fragrances that share similar characteristics, such as floral, citrus, woody, or oriental. By selecting notes from the same scent family, you can create a cohesive and harmonious fragrance. However, don't be afraid to experiment and combine notes from different families to add complexity and uniqueness to your perfume.

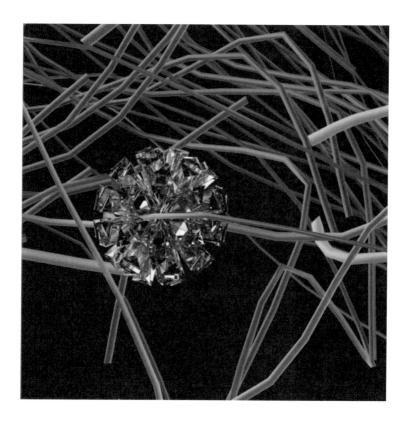

In addition to scent families, understanding scent profiles is crucial for creating balance. Scent profiles refer to the way different notes interact with each other. Some notes enhance each other, while others may clash or overpower the overall scent. By understanding the interactions between different notes, you can create a formula where each note complements and enhances the others, resulting in a well-balanced fragrance.

To achieve balance and harmony, it's also important to consider the intensity and longevity of each note. Some notes are more volatile and evaporate quickly, while others are more long-lasting. By carefully selecting and combining notes with different volatilities, you can create a perfume that unfolds beautifully and lasts throughout the day.

Lastly, experimenting with different blending techniques can also help you achieve balance and harmony in your perfume formulas. Techniques such as layering, dilution, and accords can add depth and complexity to your fragrances. Don't be afraid to experiment and trust your nose to guide you towards the perfect balance.

In conclusion, creating balance and harmony in perfume formulas is a combination of art and science. By understanding the fragrance pyramid, scent families, scent profiles, and blending techniques, you can create fragrances that are truly exceptional. Whether you're a fragrance lover, DIY enthusiast, or looking to start your own e-commerce business, mastering the art of balance and harmony in perfume making will set you on the path to creating signature scents that captivate and delight.

Experimenting with Different Blending Methods

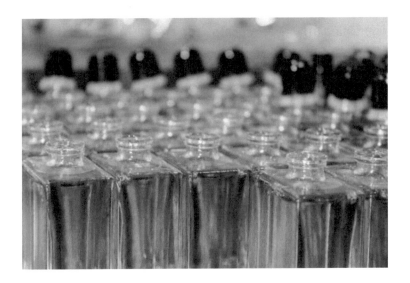

In the world of perfume making, the art of blending different scents is crucial to creating unique and captivating fragrances. As a beginner, it's essential to understand the various blending methods available to you. Experimenting with these methods will not only help you understand the science behind fragrance blending but also allow you to create your signature scents.

One popular blending method is layering. Layering involves combining multiple scents to create a complex and harmonious fragrance. This technique is perfect for those who want to create their unique scent combinations. By layering different essential oils or fragrance oils, you can create a fragrance that is entirely your own. Experiment with different combinations and proportions to find the perfect balance.

Another blending method is vintage perfume replication. If you're a fan of classic fragrances, you can try to replicate them using the original formulas or create your interpretation of these timeless scents. Vintage perfume replication requires a keen sense of smell and the ability to identify the key notes in a fragrance. By studying the composition of these classic scents and experimenting with different ingredients, you can create a fragrance that captures the essence of the past.

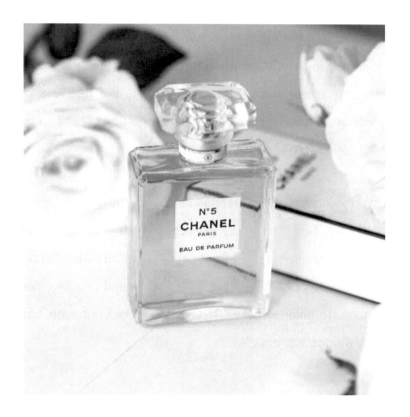

For those interested in aromatherapy fragrance blending, experimenting with different essential oils is a must. Each essential oil has its unique properties and benefits, and by combining them, you can create fragrances that promote relaxation, energy, or even focus. Experiment with different ratios to find the perfect combination for your desired effect.

Solid perfume making is another exciting blending method to explore. Solid perfumes are convenient and portable, making them a popular choice for fragrance lovers on the go. By blending essential oils with a solid base like beeswax or coconut oil, you can create your solid perfume that can be easily applied to your pulse points.

If you're interested in creating customized fragrance oils for bath and body products or scented candles, fragrance formulation is the way to go. By experimenting with different combinations of essential oils, carrier oils, and fixatives, you can create unique scents that will enhance your bath and body products or candles.

In conclusion, experimenting with different blending methods is crucial for fragrance lovers, DIY enthusiasts, and those interested in e-commerce. Whether you're looking to create your signature scent, replicate vintage perfumes, or develop customized fragrance oils, exploring the various blending methods will allow you to unleash your creativity and create fragrances that are truly one- of-a-kind. So, don't be afraid to experiment and let your nose guide you on this aromatic journey.

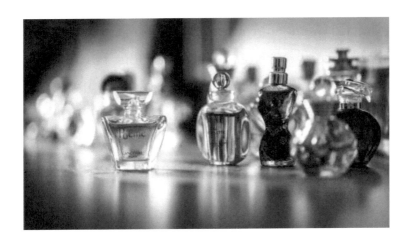

Chapter 5: Aromatherapy Fragrance Blending

Introduction to Aromatherapy

Aromatherapy has been gaining popularity among fragrance lovers, DIY enthusiasts, and those involved in the e-commerce industry. It offers a holistic and natural approach to creating fragrances and therapeutic blends using essential oils. In this subchapter, we will delve into the basics of aromatherapy, providing you with a comprehensive introduction to this captivating field.

Aromatherapy is the art and science of using essential oils extracted from aromatic plants to enhance well-being, improve mood, and promote relaxation. These essential oils are highly concentrated and possess various therapeutic properties, making them an ideal choice for creating fragrances that not only smell divine but also have a positive impact on our emotional and physical health.

Whether you are a beginner or an experienced fragrance enthusiast, understanding the principles of aromatherapy is crucial for creating unique and effective scents. In this subchapter, we will explore the different extraction methods used to obtain essential oils, as well as the various factors that influence their quality and potency.

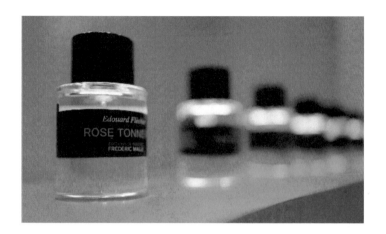

Furthermore, we will delve into the art of fragrance blending, sharing tips and techniques to help you create your signature scents. From vintage perfume replication to fragrance layering techniques, you will discover the secrets behind crafting captivating and long-lasting fragrances.

But aromatherapy is not limited to perfumes alone. We will also explore how to incorporate essential oils into other products such as scented candles, bath and body products, and even customized fragrance oils. Learn how to formulate fragrances for these mediums and elevate your DIY projects to a whole new level.

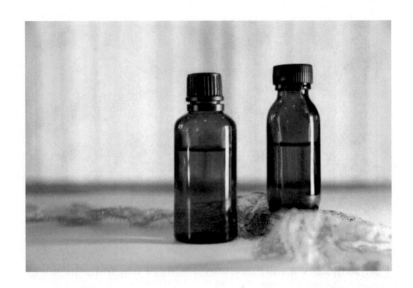

Additionally, we will touch on the topic of solid perfume making, providing step-by-step instructions on how to create compact and travel-friendly scents that you can take anywhere.

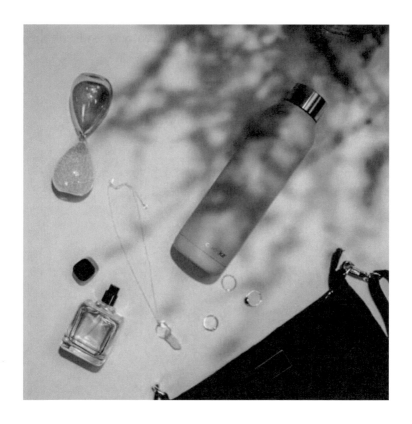

Throughout this subchapter, we will provide you with valuable insights, expert tips, and practical guidance to help you navigate the world of aromatherapy with confidence. Whether you are passionate about making fragrances for personal use or considering starting your own e-commerce business, this chapter will equip you with the essential knowledge and skills needed to succeed.

Embark on this aromatic journey, and let the captivating world of aromatherapy inspire your creativity and enhance your well-being.

Selecting Essential Oils for Aromatherapy Perfumes

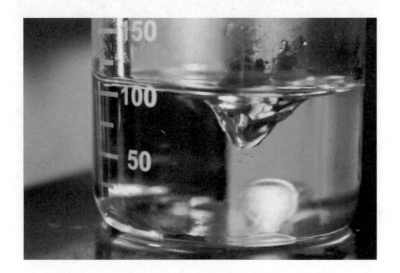

When it comes to creating your own aromatherapy perfumes, the selection of essential oils is of utmost importance. These oils not only contribute to the fragrance of your perfume but also provide therapeutic benefits that can enhance your overall well-being. In this subchapter, we will explore the process of selecting essential oils for aromatherapy perfumes, taking into consideration the preferences of fragrance lovers, DIY enthusiasts, and e-commerce sellers in the niches of perfume making, DIY natural fragrances, and more.

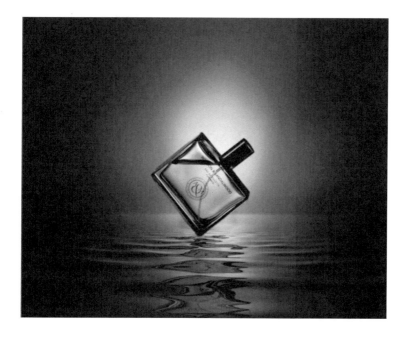

To begin, it is essential to understand the different notes in perfumery. Essential oils are classified into three categories: top notes, middle notes, and base notes. Top notes are the first impression of your perfume and typically have a light and refreshing scent. Middle notes provide the body of the fragrance and offer a harmonious balance to the perfume. Base notes are the foundation and create a long-lasting scent. When selecting essential oils for your aromatherapy perfume, it is crucial to consider a blend of these notes to create a well-rounded fragrance.

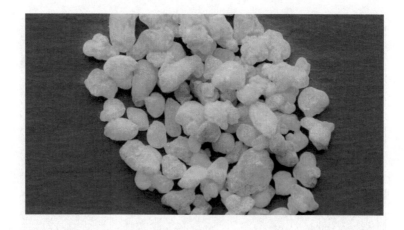

Fragrance lovers and DIY enthusiasts often prefer natural fragrances over synthetic ones. Therefore, it is advisable to choose high-quality, pure essential oils derived from plants. Some popular essential oils for aromatherapy perfumes include lavender, rose, chamomile, bergamot, and ylang-ylang. These oils not only offer delightful scents but also possess therapeutic properties such as relaxation, stress relief, and mood enhancement.

For e-commerce sellers in the fragrance niche, it is essential to consider the target market and their preferences. Vintage perfume replication and creating signature scents are popular trends. Researching the historical perfumes and their ingredients can provide insights into the essential oils that were commonly used. Additionally, experimenting with unique combinations and fragrance layering techniques can help create one-of-a-kind scents that stand out in the market.

Furthermore, as the demand for DIY natural fragrances and customized products increases, it is beneficial to explore fragrance formulation for bath and body products, scented candle making, and solid perfume making. Essential oils that are safe for skin application and have long-lasting scents are ideal for these purposes.

In conclusion, selecting essential oils for aromatherapy perfumes requires a careful consideration of the notes, preferences of fragrance lovers and DIY enthusiasts, and the specific niches such as perfume making, DIY natural fragrances, and more. By understanding the different properties and benefits of essential oils, you can create unique and therapeutic perfumes that cater to the diverse needs of your target audience.

Creating Emotional and Therapeutic Blends

In the world of fragrance, creating emotional and therapeutic blends is an art that allows individuals to express their unique style and personality. Whether you are a fragrance lover, DIY enthusiast, or involved in e-commerce, understanding how to make fragrances with emotional and therapeutic benefits can enhance your experience and elevate your creations.

Aromatherapy fragrance blending is a popular technique that combines the power of scent with the healing properties of essential oils. By carefully selecting and blending different essential oils, you can create fragrances that promote relaxation, reduce stress, or uplift the mood. For example, lavender and chamomile are known for their calming properties, while citrus oils like bergamot and lemon can boost energy and focus.

Creating signature scents is another exciting aspect of fragrance making. By experimenting with different combinations of top, middle, and base notes, you can develop a unique fragrance that reflects your personal style. Whether you prefer floral, woody, or oriental scents, the possibilities are endless. This process allows you to unleash your creativity and tailor the fragrance to your specific preferences.

Vintage perfume replication is a niche that appeals to fragrance enthusiasts and collectors. By studying historical perfume formulas and techniques, you can recreate iconic fragrances from the past. This skill allows you to experience the scents that were loved by generations before and pay homage to the art of perfumery.

Fragrance layering techniques involve combining multiple fragrances to create a complex and unique scent. This method allows you to customize your fragrance based on your mood or occasion.

It is a popular technique among fragrance lovers who enjoy experimenting with different combinations to create their own signature blend.

Solid perfume making is a fun and practical skill to have. By using a combination of carrier oils, beeswax, and fragrance oils, you can create solid perfumes that are portable and long-lasting. These perfumes can be easily applied to pulse points and are perfect for on-the-go touch-ups.

Customized fragrance oils are a valuable asset for individuals involved in e-commerce or DIY projects. By formulating your own fragrance oils, you can create unique scents for candles, bath and body products, and more. This customization allows you to differentiate your products and offer something truly special to your customers.

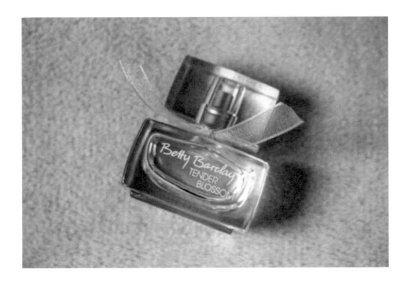

In conclusion, understanding the art of creating emotional and therapeutic blends in fragrance making opens up a world of possibilities for fragrance lovers, DIY enthusiasts, and those involved in e-commerce. Whether you are interested in making natural fragrances, exploring aromatherapy benefits, or developing signature scents, the techniques and skills discussed in this subchapter will help you on your fragrance-making journey. So, let your creativity flow and embark on a fragrant adventure that will delight your senses and bring joy to others.

Chapter 6: Crafting Signature Scents

Understanding Perfume Families and Categories

When it comes to the world of fragrances, there is a vast array of scents to explore. To help navigate this aromatic journey, it is essential to understand the concept of perfume families and categories. In this subchapter, we will delve into the different perfume families and categories, providing you with a comprehensive understanding of how fragrances are classified.

Perfume families are broad classifications that group fragrances based on their dominant scent characteristics. There are four main perfume families: floral, oriental, woody, and fresh. Each family has its unique qualities and subcategories that further define the specific scent profiles.

The floral family is the most prevalent and includes scents derived from flowers such as rose, jasmine, and lily. This family is known for its feminine and romantic qualities and is often associated with elegance and sophistication. Subcategories within the floral family include floral aldehydes, floral musks, and floral greens.

The oriental family is characterized by warm, spicy, and exotic notes such as vanilla, amber, and cinnamon. These scents evoke a sense of sensuality and mystery, making them popular choices for evening wear. Subcategories within the oriental family include soft orientals, spicy orientals, and woody orientals.

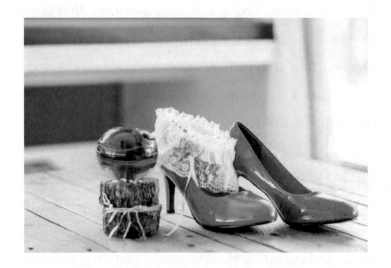

Understanding the perfume categories is equally important as it provides further specificity within each perfume family. The categories include eau de cologne, eau de toilette, eau de parfum, and perfume extract. These categories determine the concentration of fragrance oils in a perfume, with perfume extract being the most concentrated and eau de cologne being the least concentrated.

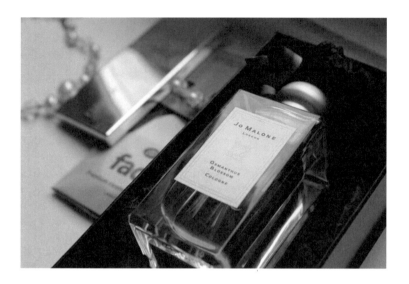

The woody family encompasses scents derived from various types of wood, such as sandalwood, cedarwood, and oud. These fragrances exude a sense of strength, grounding, and nature. Subcategories within the woody family include dry woods, mossy woods, and aromatic woods.

The fresh family is composed of scents that are light, airy, and invigorating. Citrus notes, green leaves, and aquatic elements are often found in this family. Fresh fragrances are commonly associated with a clean and revitalizing sensation. Subcategories within the fresh family include citrus, green, and aquatic.

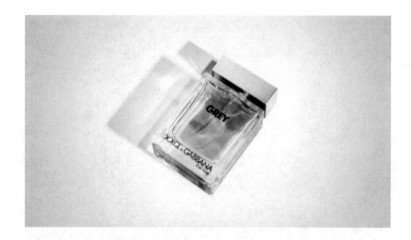

By understanding perfume families and categories, fragrance lovers, DIY enthusiasts, and e- commerce entrepreneurs can make informed choices when creating their own fragrances, exploring different scent combinations, or purchasing perfumes for themselves or their customers. This knowledge opens up a world of possibilities for creating signature scents, replicating vintage perfumes, experimenting with fragrance layering techniques, and formulating customized fragrance oils for various products such as scented candles and bath and body products.

In the following chapters, we will delve deeper into each perfume family and category, providing you with valuable insights, tips, and techniques to explore and master the art of perfume making.

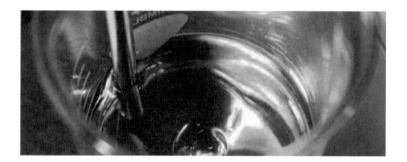

Developing Your Unique Fragrance Profile

In the world of fragrance, there is nothing more personal and intimate than creating your own signature scent. Your unique fragrance profile is a reflection of your personality, style, and preferences. It is an expression of who you are and how you want to be perceived by others. In this subchapter, we will explore the exciting journey of developing your own fragrance profile, step-by- step.

To begin, it is essential to understand the various fragrance families and notes. Fragrance families are the broad categories that scents fall into, such as floral, oriental, citrus, woody, and many more. Each family has its characteristics and evokes different emotions and moods. Understanding these families will help you in choosing the scents that resonate with you the most.

Next, consider the notes within each fragrance family. Notes are the individual scents that make up a fragrance, such as rose, vanilla, lavender, or sandalwood. These notes can be top, middle, or base notes, and they work together to create a harmonious blend. Experimenting with different notes will help you find the combinations that appeal to your senses.

Once you have a basic understanding of fragrance families and notes, it's time to start experimenting. Begin by selecting a few scents that you are drawn to and create a base blend. Start with a small quantity and gradually increase the proportions until you achieve the desired balance. Remember, fragrance creation is an art, and it may take several attempts before you find your perfect blend.

As you develop your fragrance profile, don't be afraid to think outside the box and try unconventional combinations. Mix floral and woody notes for a unique twist, or experiment with different ratios to create a scent that is entirely your own. The possibilities are endless, and the journey is part of the fun.

To enhance your fragrance profile, consider exploring fragrance layering techniques. Layering involves combining different scented products, such as body lotion, shower gel, and perfume, to create a more complex and long-lasting scent. This technique allows you to customize your fragrance to suit different occasions and moods.

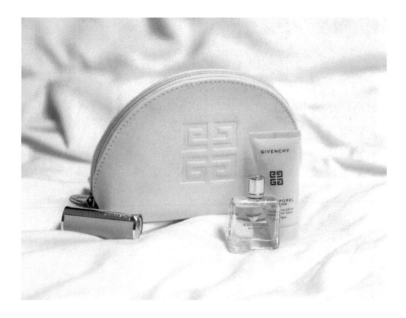

Lastly, remember that fragrance formulation is not limited to personal use. You can also explore the world of e-commerce and DIY by creating customized fragrance oils, scented candles, solid perfumes, or bath and body products. This opens up endless opportunities for creative expression and entrepreneurship.

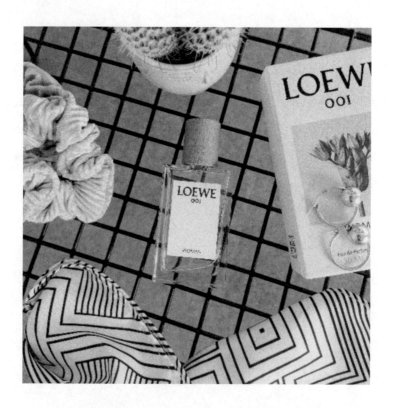

In conclusion, developing your unique fragrance profile is an exciting and personal journey. By understanding fragrance families and notes, experimenting with different combinations, and exploring fragrance layering techniques, you can create a scent that is truly your own. Whether you are a fragrance lover, DIY enthusiast, or looking to start your own e-commerce business, perfume making offers a world of possibilities. So, grab your passion for scents and embark on the delightful journey of creating your signature fragrance.

Tips for Creating Memorable and Long-lasting Scents

Creating a memorable and long-lasting scent is the goal of every perfume maker. Whether you are a fragrance lover, DIY enthusiast, or an e-commerce entrepreneur, understanding the art of creating scents that leave a lasting impression is crucial. In this subchapter, we will explore some tips and techniques that will help you achieve just that. 1. Start with a Strong Base: The foundation of a long-lasting scent lies in its base notes. Choose base ingredients such as musk, amber, or sandalwood that have a natural ability to linger on the skin and blend well with other ingredients. 2. Experiment with Blending: Don't be afraid to experiment with different combinations of essential oils and fragrance notes. Mixing different scents can create unique and memorable fragrances. Consider blending floral, citrus, and woody notes to create depth and complexity in your scent. 3.

Use High-quality Ingredients: The quality of your ingredients plays a significant role in the longevity of your scent. Invest in high-quality essential oils, fragrance oils, and carrier oils to ensure a well-rounded and long-lasting fragrance. 4. Consider the Concentration: The concentration of your perfume will determine its longevity. Higher concentrations, such as parfum or extrait de parfum, tend to last longer than eau de toilette or eau de cologne. Experiment with different concentrations to find the right balance for your fragrance. 5. Let it Mature: Patience is key when it comes to creating long-lasting scents. Allow your perfume to mature and blend for a few weeks before testing or selling. This allows the ingredients to meld together and enhances the overall longevity of the fragrance. 6. Layering Techniques: Layering different scented products can help extend the life of your fragrance.

Encourage your customers to use matching body lotions, shower gels, or solid perfumes in conjunction with your perfume to create a longer-lasting scent experience. 7. Consider the Season: Different scents perform differently in various seasons. Light and fresh scents are more suitable for summer, while warm and spicy fragrances work well in the colder months. Consider the climate and season when formulating your perfumes to ensure they last in the intended environment.

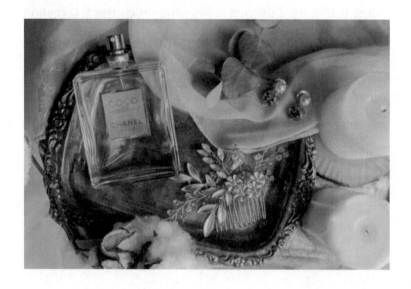

Creating memorable and long-lasting scents is an art that requires practice and experimentation. By following these tips and techniques, you can craft fragrances that leave a lasting impression on your customers. Whether you are interested in DIY natural fragrances, vintage perfume replication, or scent layering techniques, understanding the fundamentals of fragrance formulation will help you create scents that stand the test of time.

Chapter 7: Replicating Vintage Perfumes

The History and Appeal of Vintage Perfumes

Vintage perfumes have a charm and allure that is unmatched by modern fragrances. They transport us back in time, evoking memories of a bygone era and captivating our senses with their unique compositions. In this subchapter, we will explore the fascinating history and enduring appeal of vintage perfumes.

Perfume has been used for thousands of years, with ancient civilizations using it for religious ceremonies, to mask unpleasant odors, and as a symbol of status and wealth. However, it was not until the late 19th century that the modern perfume industry took shape. This era saw the birth of iconic fragrance houses such as Guerlain, Chanel, and Caron, which created some of the most enduring and beloved perfumes of all time.

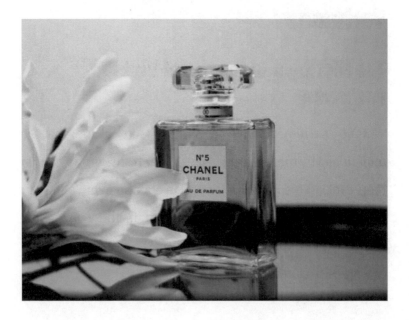

One of the reasons vintage perfumes hold such appeal is their rich and complex compositions. Unlike many modern fragrances that can be described as simple and linear, vintage perfumes are multi-layered and nuanced. They are made using a higher concentration of natural ingredients, such as precious flowers, spices, and resins, which give them a depth and complexity that is hard to replicate.

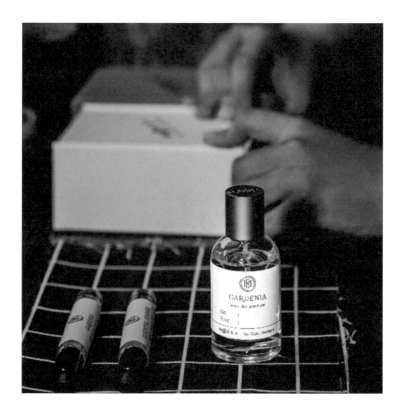

Another factor that adds to the allure of vintage perfumes is their scarcity. Many of these fragrances have been discontinued or reformulated over the years, making them rare and highly sought after by collectors and fragrance enthusiasts. Owning a vintage perfume is like owning a piece of history, a treasure that is imbued with nostalgia and a sense of timelessness.

Vintage perfumes also offer a unique olfactory experience. They have a distinctive character that sets them apart from their modern counterparts. Their vintage charm and sophistication appeal to fragrance lovers who appreciate the artistry and craftsmanship that goes into creating these timeless scents.

For DIY enthusiasts and fragrance lovers looking to recreate the magic of vintage perfumes, understanding their composition and formulation is essential. By studying the ingredients and techniques used in vintage perfumes, one can learn to replicate their unique scent profiles and create their own signature fragrances.

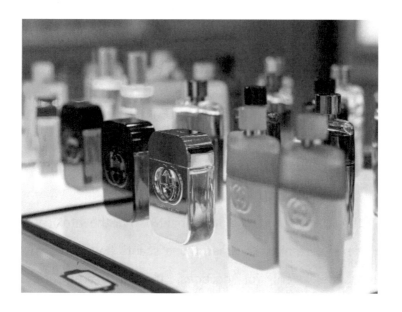

In the following chapters of this book, we will delve deeper into the world of perfume making, exploring the techniques, ingredients, and tools necessary to create your own fragrances. Whether you are interested in creating natural fragrances, experimenting with aromatherapy blends, or replicating vintage perfumes, this book will provide you with the knowledge and inspiration to embark on your fragrance-making journey.

So, join us as we explore the fascinating history and enduring appeal of vintage perfumes and discover the secrets to creating your own unique scents. Let the journey begin!

Analyzing and Replicating Classic Fragrances

In the vast world of perfumery, there is a certain allure to classic fragrances that have stood the test of time. Whether it's the timeless elegance of Chanel No. 5 or the intoxicating allure of Guerlain's Shalimar, these scents have captivated fragrance lovers for decades. If you're a fragrance enthusiast and have always wondered how these iconic perfumes are created, this subchapter is for you.

Analyzing and replicating classic fragrances is a fascinating journey that allows you to delve into the art of perfumery and gain a deeper understanding of scent composition. By studying the ingredients and notes used in these fragrances, you can begin to unravel their secrets and create your own versions that pay homage to these legendary scents.

To start, it's essential to carefully analyze the classic fragrance you want to replicate. Study its top, middle, and base notes, and try to identify the key ingredients that give it its distinct character. This process requires a keen sense of smell and a trained nose, but with practice, you can develop these skills.

Once you have familiarized yourself with the fragrance, it's time to start the replication process. Begin by selecting high-quality essential oils, absolutes, and fragrance oils that closely resemble the notes of the original perfume. Experiment with different combinations and proportions until you achieve a scent that closely resembles the classic fragrance you're aiming to replicate.

Remember, replicating a classic fragrance doesn't mean creating an exact copy. It's about capturing the essence and feel of the original scent while adding your own unique twist. This is where your creativity as a fragrance lover and DIY enthusiast shines through. Don't be afraid to experiment and explore different scent combinations to create your own signature version of the classic fragrance.

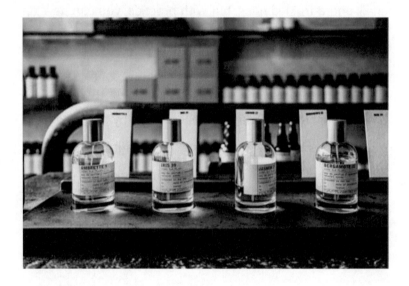

Analyzing and replicating classic fragrances is not only a rewarding hobby but also a useful skill for those interested in e-commerce. With the growing popularity of DIY natural fragrances and customized fragrance oils, being able to replicate and create unique scents can open up a world of opportunities in the fragrance industry.

So, if you're passionate about perfume making and have a love for classic fragrances, dive into the art of analyzing and replicating these scents. Unlock the secrets of the great perfumers of the past, and create your own unique fragrances that will captivate and delight others in the world of fragrance.

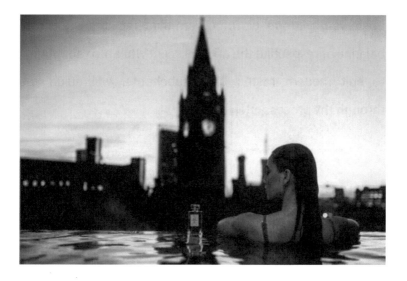

Preserving and Modernizing Vintage Perfume Formulas

Vintage perfumes hold a special place in the hearts of fragrance lovers. The unique scents and exquisite craftsmanship of these timeless classics have stood the test of time. As a DIY enthusiast or someone in the e-commerce fragrance industry, you may be interested in learning how to preserve and modernize vintage perfume formulas.

Preserving vintage perfume formulas requires a delicate balance of respecting the original scent while also adapting it to suit modern tastes. This subchapter will guide you through the process, step by step.

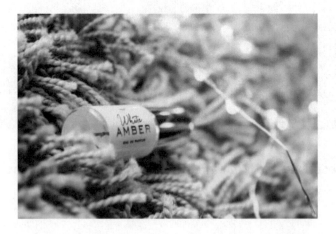

First, it's important to research and understand the original formula. Vintage perfume formulas often consist of a unique blend of essential oils, absolutes, and synthetic compounds. By studying the ingredients and ratios used, you can gain insight into the fragrance's composition and recreate it faithfully.

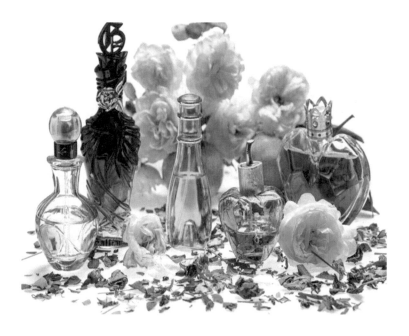

Once you have a grasp on the original formula, it's time to evaluate its relevance in today's market. Consider the preferences of your target audience — what scents are trending, and what modifications can be made to appeal to their tastes? This is where the modernization aspect comes into play.

To modernize a vintage perfume formula, you can experiment with adding contemporary notes or adjusting the concentrations of certain ingredients. This ensures that the fragrance retains its classic charm while also appealing to a wider range of consumers.

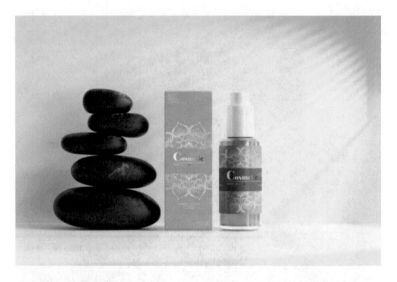

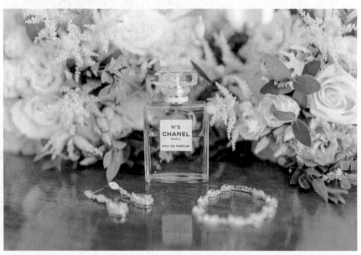

It's important to note that vintage perfume formulas often contain ingredients that are now restricted or banned due to safety concerns. In such cases, you will need to find suitable alternatives or omit those ingredients altogether. This is where your expertise in fragrance formulation comes into play.

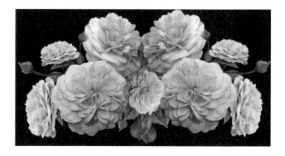

Once you have preserved and modernized the vintage perfume formula, you can explore various applications for it. Fragrance layering techniques, solid perfume making, customized fragrance oils, scented candle making, and fragrance formulation for bath and body products are all potential avenues to showcase your revived creation.

In conclusion, preserving and modernizing vintage perfume formulas is a rewarding journey that combines the art of perfumery with the needs and desires of today's fragrance lovers. By respecting the original formula while adapting it to suit modern tastes, you can create something truly special – a fragrance that pays homage to the past while capturing the spirit of the present.

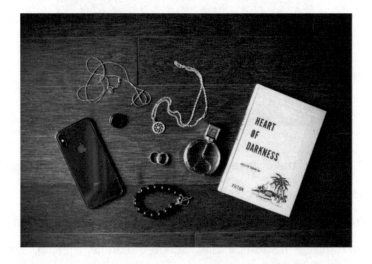

Chapter 8: Fragrance Layering Techniques

Introduction to Fragrance Layering

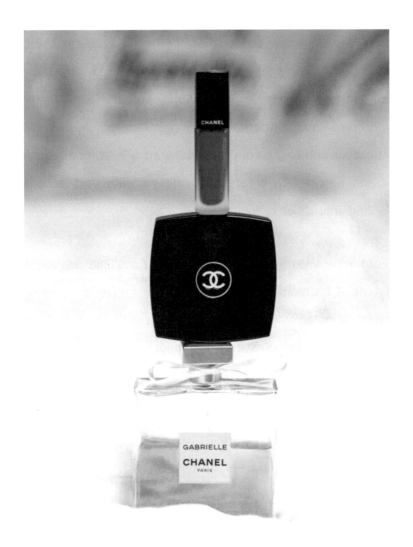

In the world of perfumery, there is an art to creating a unique and personalized scent that perfectly captures your individuality. One technique that has gained popularity among fragrance lovers, DIY enthusiasts, and e-commerce entrepreneurs is fragrance layering. This subchapter will introduce you to the concept of fragrance layering and how it can be used to create captivating scents that leave a lasting impression.

Fragrance layering involves combining multiple scents to create a harmonious and complex fragrance. By layering different notes, you can enhance the longevity and depth of a scent, as well as create a truly one-of-a-kind fragrance that reflects your personality and style.

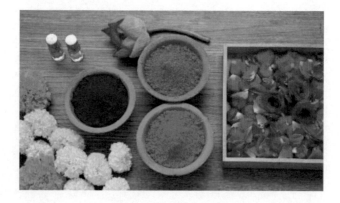

For DIY enthusiasts, fragrance layering opens up a world of possibilities. With a wide variety of essential oils, fragrance oils, and natural ingredients at your disposal, you can experiment with different combinations to create your own signature scents. Whether you're looking to replicate a vintage perfume, create a customized fragrance oil, or formulate scents for bath and body products, fragrance layering allows you to unleash your creativity and craft unique aromas that stand out from the crowd.

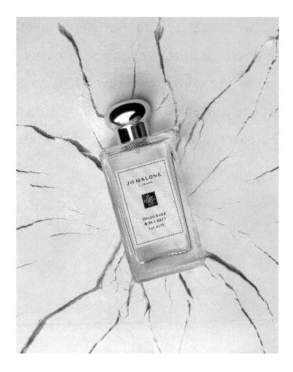

Aromatherapy fragrance blending is another niche where fragrance layering can be particularly beneficial. By combining essential oils known for their therapeutic properties, you can create fragrances that not only smell amazing but also provide a range of emotional and physical benefits. From relaxation and stress relief to energizing and uplifting effects, the possibilities are endless.

In addition to its creative potential, fragrance layering also offers practical advantages. For those interested in e-commerce, fragrance layering can be a great way to differentiate your products and offer customers a unique experience. By developing your own fragrance layering techniques, you can create scented candles, solid perfumes, and other products that stand out in a crowded market.

This subchapter will guide you through the basics of fragrance layering, including how to choose complementary notes, understanding fragrance families, and the dos and don'ts of layering different scents. We will also explore advanced techniques such as accords and blending ratios, allowing you to take your fragrance layering skills to the next level.

Whether you're a fragrance lover, DIY enthusiast, or e-commerce entrepreneur, fragrance layering is a valuable technique to add to your arsenal. Join us on this olfactory journey as we dive into the world of fragrance layering and discover the endless possibilities it holds for creating captivating and unique scents.

Complementary and Contrasting Scent Pairings

In the world of perfume making, understanding how different scents interact with each other is essential to creating well-balanced and captivating fragrances. Complementary and contrasting scent pairings are two techniques that can help you achieve the desired effect in your scent compositions. Whether you are a fragrance lover, a DIY enthusiast, or an e-commerce entrepreneur looking to dive into the world of perfume making, mastering these techniques is crucial.

Complementary scent pairings involve combining fragrances that share similar characteristics or notes. This technique creates a harmonious blend that enhances the overall scent profile. For example, if you are working with a floral fragrance, you can complement it with another floral note that has a slightly different character, such as a rose and jasmine combination. This pairing creates a beautiful bouquet-like scent that is both sophisticated and alluring. Complementary pairings can also be achieved by combining different notes within the same fragrance family, such as citrus and woody or oriental and spicy.

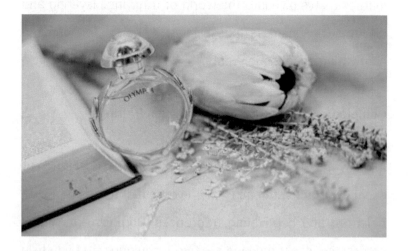

On the other hand, contrasting scent pairings involve combining fragrances that have opposing characteristics or notes. This technique creates a dynamic and intriguing scent profile that captivates the senses. For instance, pairing a fresh and zesty citrus note with a warm and sensual vanilla note

can create a unique and unexpected fragrance that is both refreshing and comforting. Contrasting pairings can also be achieved by combining notes from different fragrance families, such as floral and aquatic or fruity and woody.

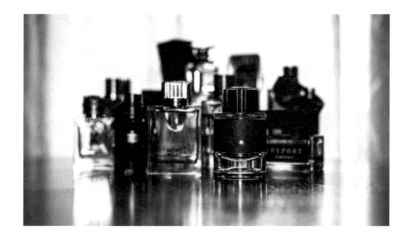

Experimenting with complementary and contrasting scent pairings allows you to create signature scents that reflect your personal style and taste. It also opens up endless possibilities for creating unique fragrances that stand out in the market. Whether you are interested in vintage perfume replication, fragrance layering techniques, or solid perfume making, mastering these scent pairing techniques is essential.

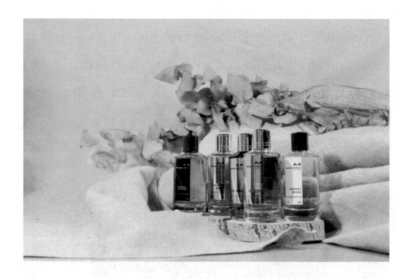

For those interested in DIY natural fragrances, aromatherapy fragrance blending, or creating customized fragrance oils for bath and body products, understanding complementary and contrasting scent pairings is equally important. These techniques can help you create well-balanced and therapeutic blends that enhance your well-being and provide a sensory experience.

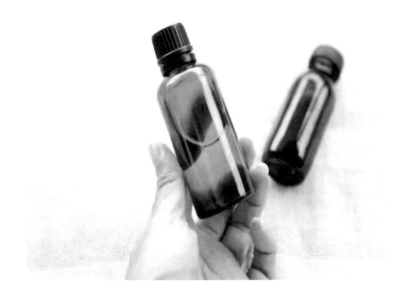

In conclusion, whether you are a fragrance lover, a DIY enthusiast, or an e-commerce entrepreneur, understanding complementary and contrasting scent pairings is crucial in the world of perfume making. These techniques allow you to create harmonious and captivating fragrances that reflect your personal style and taste. So, grab your essential oils, experiment with different combinations, and embark on a fragrant journey of discovery and creativity.

Layering Fragrances for Different Occasions

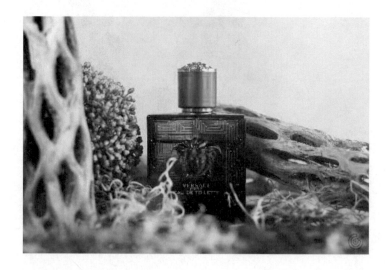

Creating the perfect fragrance for any occasion can be a daunting task, especially if you are new to the world of perfume making. However, with a little knowledge and experimentation, you can easily learn how to layer fragrances to suit different occasions. In this subchapter, we will explore various techniques and tips for blending scents to create unique and captivating fragrances.

Whether you are a fragrance lover, DIY enthusiast, or involved in e-commerce, understanding how to make fragrances that cater to different occasions is essential. From creating signature scents to replicating vintage perfumes, this subchapter will cover it all.

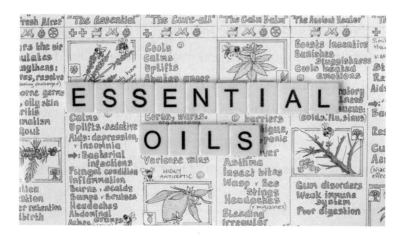

One technique for layering fragrances is to start with a base scent, such as a woody or musky fragrance, and then add complementary top and middle notes. For example, if you are creating a fragrance for a romantic evening, you might start with a warm, sensual base note like vanilla or sandalwood. To add depth and complexity, you can then layer on top notes like rose or jasmine, which are known for their romantic and seductive qualities. Finally, you can balance the fragrance by adding middle notes like lavender or bergamot, which provide a fresh and calming effect.

Another technique is to create a customized fragrance oil by blending different essential oils and carrier oils. This allows you to create a unique scent that is tailored to your personal preferences and the occasion. For example, if you are attending a formal event, you might choose to blend floral and citrus essential oils to create a light and refreshing fragrance. On the other hand, if you are going for a casual outing, you might opt for a blend of fruity and herbal essential oils to create a more vibrant and energetic scent.

In addition to perfume making, fragrance layering techniques can also be applied to other products like solid perfumes, scented candles, and bath and body products. By understanding the different notes and their effects, you can create a cohesive scent experience across all these products, enhancing the overall ambiance and mood.

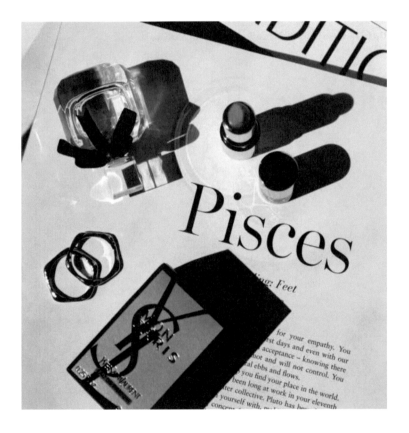

In conclusion, layering fragrances for different occasions is a skill that can be honed with practice and experimentation. By understanding the various techniques and tips mentioned in this subchapter, fragrance lovers, DIY enthusiasts, and e-commerce professionals can create unique, customized fragrances that cater to their specific niche. So go ahead, unleash your creativity, and start blending scents to create captivating fragrances for any occasion.

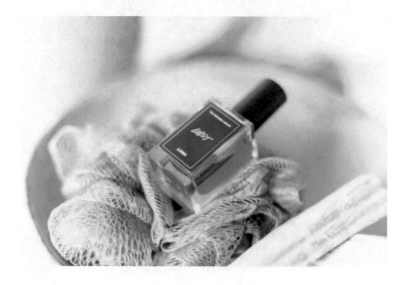

Chapter 9: Solid Perfume Making

Benefits and Advantages of Solid Perfumes

Solid perfumes have gained immense popularity in recent years, and for good reason. These innovative fragrances offer a range of benefits and advantages that make them a favorite among fragrance lovers, DIY enthusiasts, and e-commerce businesses. In this subchapter, we will explore the numerous reasons why solid perfumes should be a part of every fragrance lover's collection. 1. Portability: One of the standout advantages of solid perfumes is their compact size and portability. Unlike traditional liquid perfumes, solid perfumes come in small, convenient containers that can easily fit in your pocket or purse. This makes them perfect for on-the-go fragrance touch-ups, travel, or simply keeping your signature scent close at hand. 2. Long-lasting: Solid perfumes are known for their long-lasting scent.

The waxy base of these perfumes helps to slow down the evaporation process, allowing the fragrance to stay on the skin for extended periods. This means you can enjoy your favorite scent throughout the day without the need for frequent reapplication. 3. Precise application: Solid perfumes offer precise application, allowing you to control the amount of fragrance you apply. The solid format allows for targeted application to pulse points, ensuring that the scent is concentrated in the areas you desire. This precision also helps in preventing wastage and allows you to make the most of your perfume. 4. Versatility: Solid perfumes are incredibly versatile and can be used in various ways.

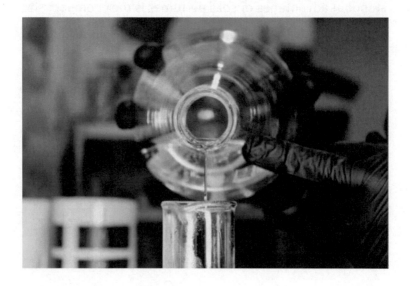

Besides applying them directly on the skin, they can be used to add fragrance to other products such as candles, bath and body products, or even as a base for creating customized fragrance oils.

The possibilities are endless, making solid perfumes a must-have for those interested in DIY fragrance projects. 5. Natural and skin-friendly: Many solid perfumes are made from natural ingredients, making them a great choice for those with sensitive skin or those who prefer using products with fewer synthetic chemicals. These perfumes are often formulated with nourishing oils and butters that not only impart a beautiful fragrance but also moisturize the skin.

In conclusion, solid perfumes offer a range of benefits and advantages that make them a valuable addition to any fragrance lover's collection. Their portability, long-lasting scent, precise application, versatility, and skin-friendly formulations make them a popular choice among DIY enthusiasts, e- commerce businesses, and anyone interested in creating their own signature scents. Whether you are a fragrance lover, a DIY enthusiast, or an e-commerce entrepreneur, exploring the world of solid perfumes is sure to enhance your fragrance experience and open up new creative possibilities.

Choosing the Right Base for Solid Perfumes

Creating your own solid perfume can be a rewarding and enjoyable experience. Not only does it allow you to tailor your fragrance to your personal preferences, but it also gives you the opportunity to experiment with different base materials. The base of your solid perfume is crucial, as it serves as the foundation for the scent and determines its longevity and texture.

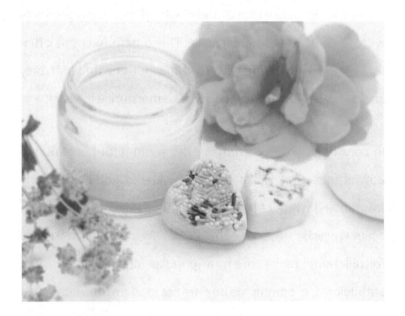

When it comes to selecting the right base for your solid perfumes, there are several factors to consider. First and foremost, you need a base that is solid at room temperature but melts upon contact with the skin, releasing the fragrance. Beeswax is a popular choice for solid perfumes, as it provides a firm texture and has a low melting point, making it easy to apply. It also has the added benefit of being all-natural and offering a subtle honey-like scent.

Another option for a solid perfume base is shea butter. Known for its moisturizing properties, shea butter creates a creamy texture that melts smoothly onto the skin. It is an excellent choice for those with dry or sensitive skin, as it nourishes and hydrates while delivering the fragrance.

If you prefer a vegan or plant-based alternative, candelilla wax is a great option. Derived from the candelilla shrub, this wax creates a firm texture and has a high melting point, ensuring that your solid perfume will stay intact even in warmer climates.

For those looking for a more luxurious and silky texture, consider using cocoa butter as your base. Cocoa butter is not only rich in antioxidants but also has a delightful chocolate aroma. Its smooth and velvety consistency makes it a popular choice for solid perfumes.

Lastly, if you want to experiment with different textures and consistencies, consider combining different bases. For example, mixing beeswax with shea butter will create a softer and more spreadable perfume, while adding a touch of cocoa butter will give it a creamier texture.

In conclusion, choosing the right base for your solid perfumes is essential for creating a long-lasting and enjoyable fragrance. Whether you opt for beeswax, shea butter, candelilla wax, cocoa butter, or a combination of these, each base offers its unique benefits and characteristics. Experiment with different bases to find the one that suits your preferences and skin type best. Happy perfume making!

Creating Solid Perfume Blends and Recipes

Solid perfumes are a fantastic option for fragrance lovers who prefer a more subtle and portable way to enjoy their favorite scents. In this subchapter, we will delve into the art of creating solid perfume blends and recipes, providing step-by-step instructions for beginners to master this craft.

To make solid perfumes, you will need a few essential ingredients: a base, fragrance oils or essential oils, and optional additives for texture and longevity. For the base, you can choose from beeswax, shea butter, cocoa butter, or a combination of these. Each base has its unique properties, so feel free to experiment and find the one that suits your preferences.

Once you have chosen your base, it's time to select the fragrance oils or essential oils for your blend. This is where your creativity can shine! Whether you want to create a floral, woody, or citrusy scent, there are countless combinations to explore. Consider blending different notes, such as lavender and bergamot for a calming aroma or patchouli and vanilla for a sensual fragrance.

Chapter 10: Customized Fragrance Oils

To achieve the desired texture and longevity, you can add optional ingredients such as jojoba oil or coconut oil. These oils not only enhance the moisturizing properties of your solid perfume but also help the fragrance to linger on the skin for a longer time. Remember to experiment with different ratios to find the perfect balance for your blend.

Once you have gathered all your ingredients, it's time to start creating your solid perfume. Begin by melting the base in a double boiler or microwave, making sure to stir it gently until it reaches a smooth consistency. Once melted, add your chosen fragrance oils or essential oils, adjusting the amount based on your desired strength.

Pour the mixture into small containers or molds, allowing it to cool and solidify. You can choose from various options, such as compact tins, locket necklaces, or even lip balm tubes for easy application. Remember to label your creations with the names of the scents used, allowing you to recreate your favorite blends in the future.

Creating solid perfume blends and recipes is an enjoyable and rewarding process that allows you to customize your own signature scents. It is also an excellent option for DIY enthusiasts and e- commerce sellers looking to offer unique and natural fragrance products. So, grab your ingredients, unleash your creativity, and start crafting your own solid perfumes today!

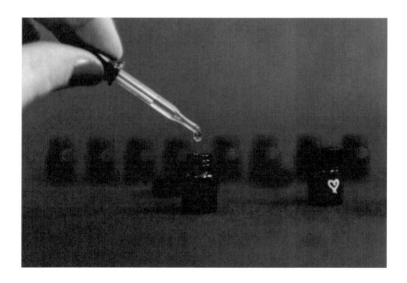

Introduction to Fragrance Oils

Fragrance oils play a crucial role in the world of perfumery and fragrance creation. Whether you are a fragrance lover, a DIY enthusiast, or an e-commerce entrepreneur looking to dive into the world of perfume making, understanding the basics of fragrance oils is essential. In this subchapter, we will introduce you to the captivating world of fragrance oils, exploring their significance, types, and applications.

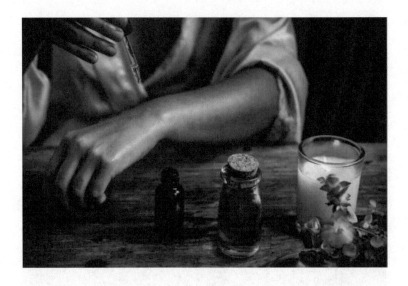

Fragrance oils are concentrated aromatic compounds that are used to add scent to various products, including perfumes, candles, bath and body products, and even household cleaners. These oils are carefully crafted using a blend of natural and synthetic ingredients to create unique and captivating scents. Unlike essential oils, fragrance oils are specifically formulated to provide a long-lasting and consistent aroma, making them ideal for use in perfumes and other fragranced products.

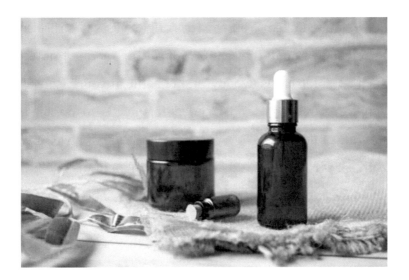

There are various types of fragrance oils available, each with its own unique characteristics and applications. Natural fragrance oils are derived from plant-based sources, such as flowers, fruits, and spices, and they provide a true-to-nature scent. On the other hand, synthetic fragrance oils are created in a lab and offer a wide range of scents that may not be found in nature. These synthetic oils allow perfumers to create complex and innovative fragrances that cater to different preferences and moods.

For fragrance lovers, fragrance oils offer endless possibilities for creating signature scents. With a wide range of notes, such as floral, citrus, woody, and oriental, at your disposal, you can experiment and blend different oils to design a fragrance that reflects your personality and style. DIY enthusiasts can also explore the art of perfume making using fragrance oils, learning the techniques of blending and layering to create unique and customized fragrances.

Fragrance oils are not limited to perfumes alone. They can be used in various other applications, such as scented candle making, where they add a delightful aroma to your living space. Additionally, fragrance oils can be incorporated into bath and body products, allowing you to create personalized scented lotions, soaps, and bath bombs.

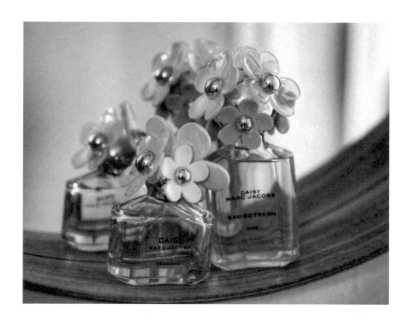

Whether you are interested in vintage perfume replication, aromatherapy fragrance blending, or simply want to learn the art of creating your own fragrances, understanding the world of fragrance oils is a vital first step. In the chapters that follow, we will delve deeper into the intricacies of fragrance oils, learning about their formulation, storage, and how to incorporate them into different products. Get ready to embark on a fragrant journey, where you will unlock the secrets of scent and create captivating fragrances that leave a lasting impression.

Blending Essential Oils with Carrier Oils

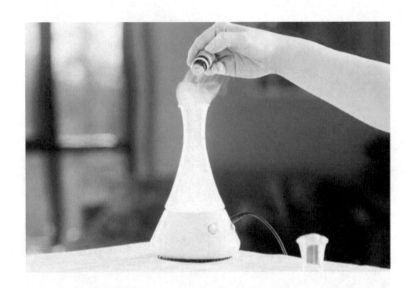

In the world of perfume making, the art of blending essential oils with carrier oils is an essential skill that every fragrance lover should master. Whether you are a DIY enthusiast, an e-commerce entrepreneur, or simply someone who wants to create their own signature scent, understanding the principles of blending these oils is crucial.

Carrier oils, also known as base oils, are neutral oils that dilute and carry the potent essential oils, allowing them to be safely applied to the skin. They act as a medium to enhance the longevity and diffusion of the fragrance. Some popular carrier oils include jojoba oil, sweet almond oil, grapeseed oil, and coconut oil.

When it comes to blending essential oils with carrier oils, there are a few key considerations to keep in mind. Firstly, you need to understand the properties of each essential oil and carrier oil you are

using. Different oils have different scent profiles, viscosities, and absorption rates. By understanding these characteristics, you can create well-balanced blends that are harmonious and long-lasting.

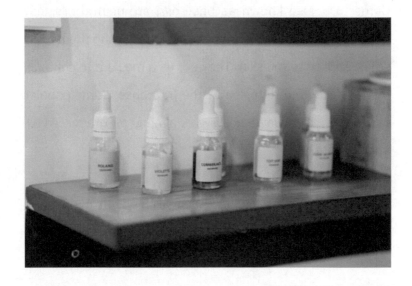

Secondly, it's important to consider the intended use of your fragrance blend. Are you creating a perfume for personal use, or are you formulating a fragrance for a scented candle? Each application requires a different approach to blending. For example, if you are creating a perfume, you may want to focus on top, middle, and base notes to create a complex and layered scent experience. On the other hand, if you are making a scented candle, you might want to prioritize the longevity and diffusion of the fragrance, using carrier oils that have a higher flashpoint.

Lastly, experimentation is key. Blending essential oils with carrier oils is a creative process that requires trial and error. Don't be afraid to mix different oils together, test them on your skin or in various products, and make adjustments until you achieve the desired result.

In this chapter, we will explore various blending techniques, such as fragrance layering, vintage perfume replication, and solid perfume making. We will also delve into the world of customized fragrance oils and fragrance formulation for bath and body products. Whether you are a beginner or an experienced fragrance enthusiast, this chapter will equip you with the knowledge and skills to create beautiful and unique fragrances that captivate the senses. Get ready to embark on a scented journey of self-expression and creativity!

Creating Personalized Fragrance Oil Blends

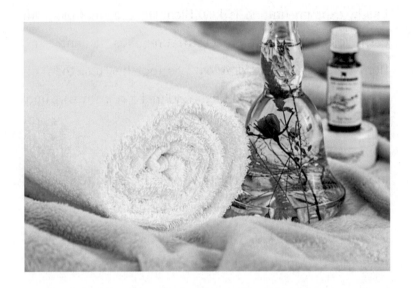

In the world of perfumery, there is nothing quite as satisfying as creating your own unique fragrance. The ability to craft a scent that is perfectly tailored to your preferences is a skill that every fragrance lover should possess. In this subchapter, we will explore the art of creating personalized fragrance oil blends, a technique that allows you to mix and match different oils to create your own signature scent.

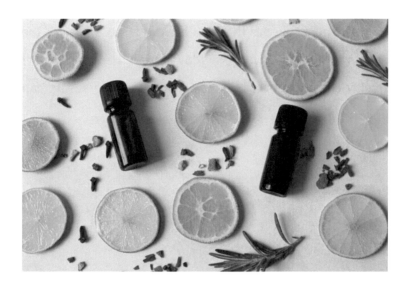

Before we delve into the process of creating personalized fragrance oil blends, it is important to understand the basics of fragrance notes. Fragrances are typically made up of three main notes: top, middle, and base. Top notes are the first scents you smell when you apply a fragrance, and they tend to be fresh and light. Middle notes, on the other hand, are the heart of the fragrance and provide depth and complexity. Finally, base notes are the scents that linger on the skin for hours, providing a lasting impression.

To begin creating your personalized fragrance oil blend, start by selecting a few oils that you are drawn to. Consider the scents that you enjoy in everyday life, such as the smell of freshly cut grass or a bouquet of roses. These scents can serve as inspiration for your blend.

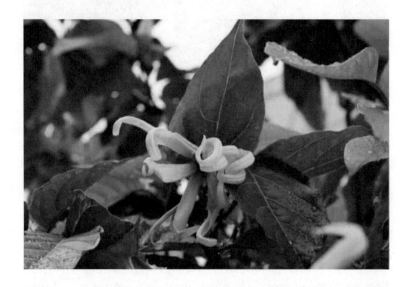

Once you have chosen your oils, it's time to start experimenting. Begin by combining a few drops of each oil in a small glass bottle. Shake the bottle gently to mix the oils together and then let it sit for a few hours to allow the scents to blend. After a few hours, give the blend a sniff and see how you like it. If it's not quite right, you can always adjust the ratios of the oils or add in a new one to create a more balanced scent.

As you continue to experiment with different oils and combinations, you will start to develop a better understanding of how different scents work together. You may even discover a few unexpected combinations that you absolutely love. Remember, fragrance blending is a highly personal and subjective process, so trust your instincts and have fun with it.

Creating personalized fragrance oil blends is not only a great way to express your creativity, but it also allows you to create scents that are truly unique to you. Whether you are interested in DIY natural fragrances, perfume making for beginners, or simply enjoy the art of fragrance blending, this technique is sure to enhance your fragrance journey. So, grab your favorite oils and start creating your signature scent today!

Chapter II: Scented Candle Making

Basics of Candle Making

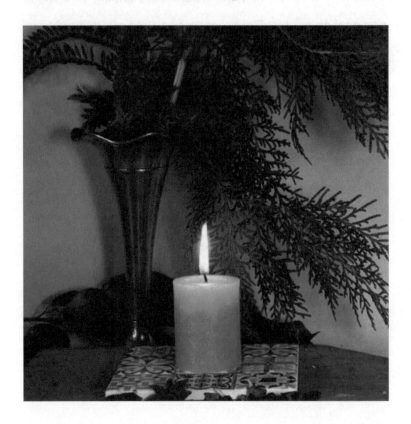

Candle making is a fascinating craft that allows you to create beautiful and fragrant candles right in the comfort of your own home. Whether you're a fragrance lover, DIY enthusiast, or looking to explore the world of e-commerce, learning the basics of candle making is essential. In this subchapter, we will take you through the step-by-step process of creating your own scented candles, giving you the tools and knowledge to start your candle-making journey.

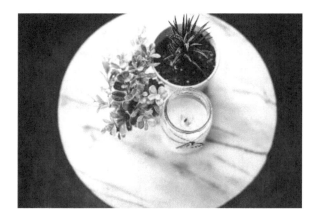

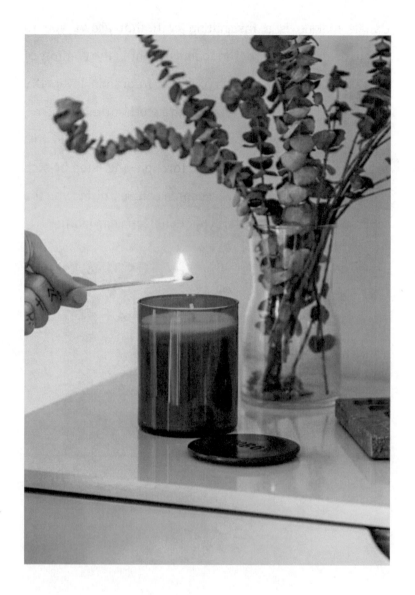

To begin, let's talk about the materials you'll need. The primary components of a candle are wax, wick, fragrance oil, and a container. There are various types of waxes to choose from, including soy, beeswax, and paraffin. Each has its own unique properties, so it's important to select the one that best suits your needs. The wick should be made of cotton or hemp, and the fragrance oil should be specifically designed for candle making to ensure proper scent throw.

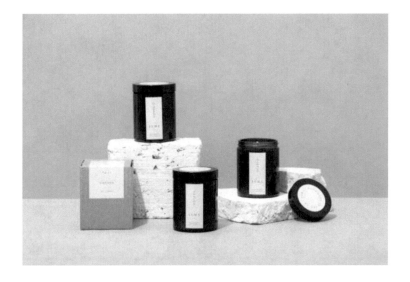

Next, we'll discuss the different candle-making techniques. The most common method is the container candle method, where the wax is melted and poured into a container with the wick placed in the center. This technique is beginner-friendly and allows for endless creativity in terms of container choices and candle designs. We will also touch on other techniques, such as pillar candles and taper candles, for those looking to expand their candle-making repertoire.

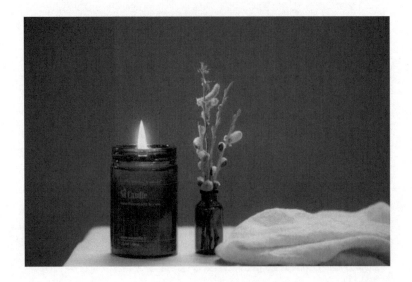

Once you have mastered the basics, we'll dive into the world of fragrance blending. Just like in perfume making, creating unique scents for your candles is a thrilling process. We'll explore different fragrance notes, blending techniques, and tips for achieving a balanced and harmonious aroma in your candles. You'll learn how to create signature scents, replicate vintage perfumes, and even layer fragrances to add complexity to your creations.

Lastly, we'll discuss the importance of proper fragrance formulation for bath and body products. If you're interested in expanding your business or simply want to create complementary products, understanding the basics of fragrance formulation is crucial. We'll explore how to create customized fragrance oils and how to incorporate them into various bath and body products, such as soaps, lotions, and bath bombs.

Whether you're a beginner looking to start your candle-making journey or a fragrance lover seeking to expand your knowledge, the basics of candle making are essential. Join us as we explore the art of creating scented candles and discover the endless possibilities of fragrance blending. Get ready to unleash your creativity and bring the warmth and beauty of candles into your life.

Selecting Fragrances for Candles

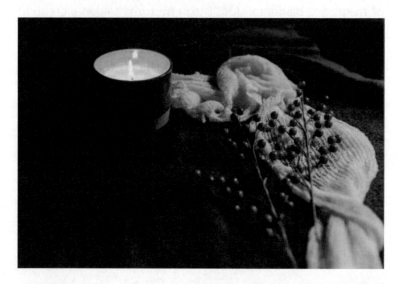

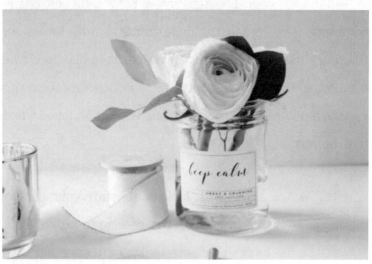

Candles have long been a popular way to create ambiance and add a touch of fragrance to any space. Whether you are a fragrance lover, a DIY enthusiast, or an e-commerce entrepreneur looking to expand your product line, selecting the right fragrances for your candles is essential to create a captivating sensory experience. In this subchapter, we will explore the factors to consider when choosing fragrances for candles and provide useful tips and techniques to help you create unique and appealing scents.

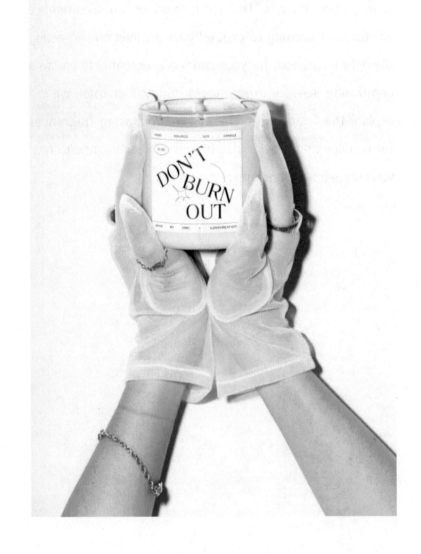

When it comes to selecting fragrances for candles, it is important to consider the intended purpose and target audience. For fragrance lovers, experimenting with different scent combinations can be a fun and rewarding experience. DIY enthusiasts may be interested in creating natural fragrances to align with their eco-friendly lifestyle. And e-commerce entrepreneurs can benefit from understanding the preferences and trends in the market to cater to their customer base effectively.

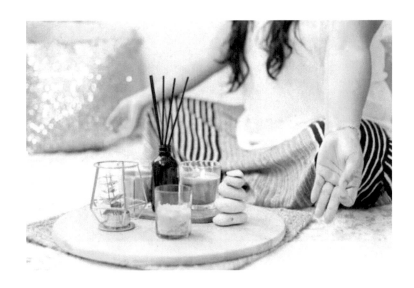

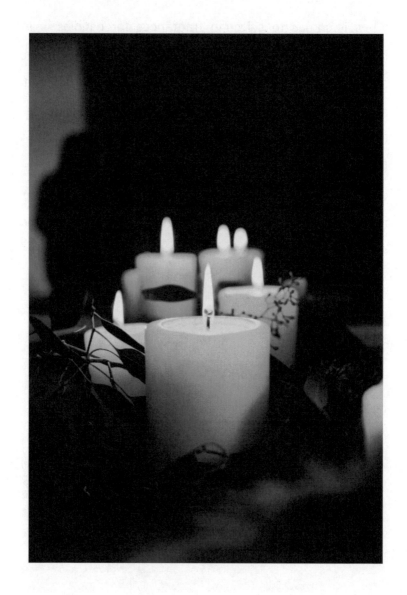

One approach to fragrance selection is to consider the desired mood or theme for your candles. Aromatherapy fragrance blending techniques can help you create scents that promote relaxation, stress relief, or focus. For those interested in creating signature scents, understanding fragrance families and notes is crucial. You can combine different fragrance oils to achieve a harmonious blend that represents your personal style or brand.

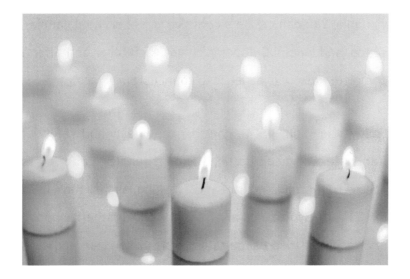

If you are fascinated by vintage perfumes, replicating their scents in candles can be a nostalgic and unique offering. Fragrance layering techniques can help you achieve depth and complexity in your candle scents, just like in perfumery. Additionally, solid perfume making techniques can be adapted to create scented candles with a unique texture and long-lasting fragrance.

For those interested in customization, understanding fragrance formulation for bath and body products can be valuable. You can create a cohesive line of scented candles, soaps, and lotions that complement each other and offer a complete sensory experience to your customers.

Lastly, it is important to consider the quality and safety of fragrance oils when selecting them for candles. Look for oils specifically formulated for candle making, as they have been tested for performance and safety. Consider the flashpoint and recommended usage rates to ensure a clean and even burn.

In conclusion, selecting fragrances for candles is an art that requires careful consideration of the intended purpose, target audience, and desired mood or theme. By understanding various techniques and trends, you can create captivating scents that not only enhance the ambiance but also offer a unique sensory experience to your customers.

Techniques for Incorporating Fragrances into Candles

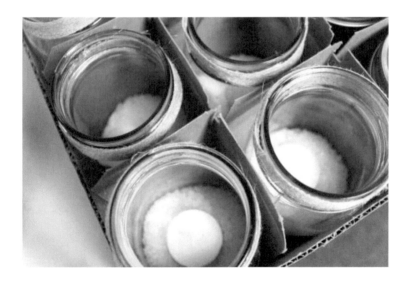

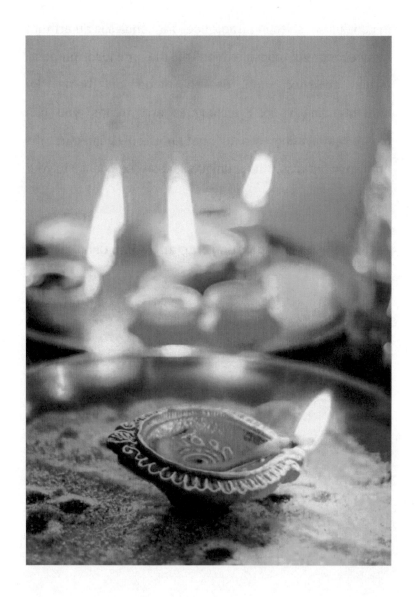

Introduction: Candles have been used for centuries to create ambiance, set a mood, and add a touch of luxury to any space. One of the key factors that make candles so special is their fragrance. The scent of a candle can transport you to a different time or place, evoke emotions, and enhance relaxation. This subchapter explores various techniques for incorporating fragrances into candles, allowing you to create personalized scents that cater to your unique preferences. 1. Choosing the Right Fragrance: The first step in creating scented candles is selecting the fragrance oils or essential oils that will be used. Consider the mood you want to create, the purpose of the candle, and the preferences of your target audience. Experiment with different combinations and ratios to find the perfect scent. 2.

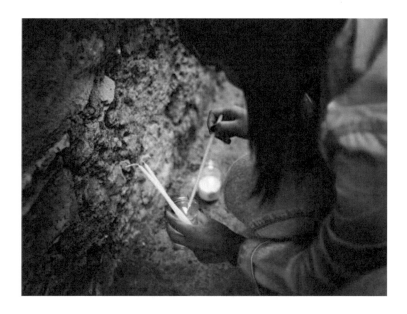

Measuring Fragrance Oils: It's crucial to measure fragrance oils accurately to ensure a well-balanced scent.

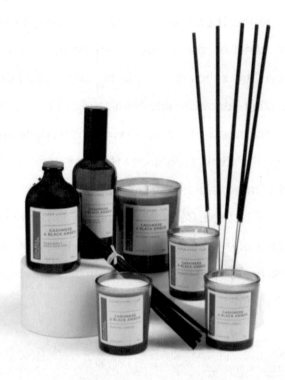

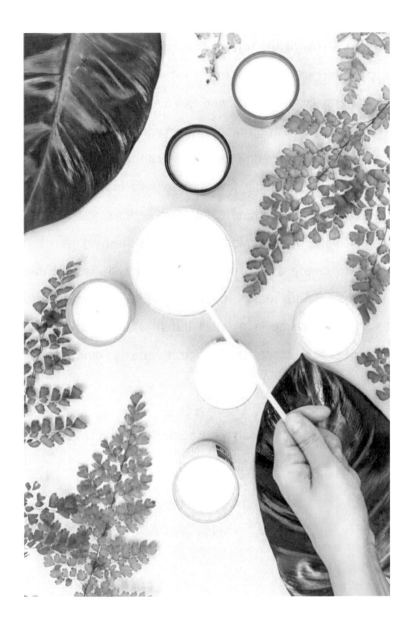

Use a digital scale to measure the correct amount, typically around 6-10% of the total wax weight. Be cautious not to exceed the recommended usage rate to avoid overpowering or potentially harmful candles. 3. Fragrance Layering Techniques: For fragrance lovers who want to create complex scents, layering techniques can be employed. This involves using multiple fragrance oils to create a unique blend. Experiment with different combinations, starting with a base note, adding middle notes, and finishing with top notes to create a well-rounded fragrance. 4. Testing and Adjusting: Before mass-producing candles, it's essential to test the fragrance in a small batch. This allows you to evaluate the scent throw, burn quality, and overall performance.

Adjust the fragrance load if necessary, ensuring the scent is neither too weak nor overwhelming.

5. Scented Candle Making Tips: To ensure the fragrance is evenly distributed throughout the candle, stir the melted wax and fragrance oil mixture thoroughly. Consider using fragrance enhancers, such as candle additives or fixatives, to improve scent retention. Additionally, choose the appropriate wick size and type to optimize burn performance.

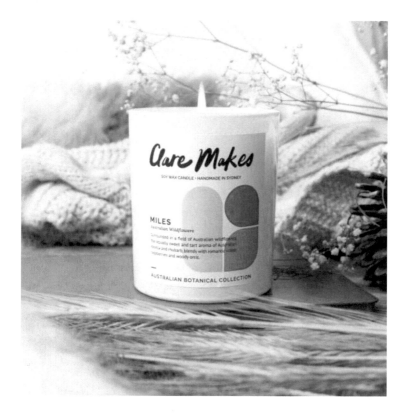

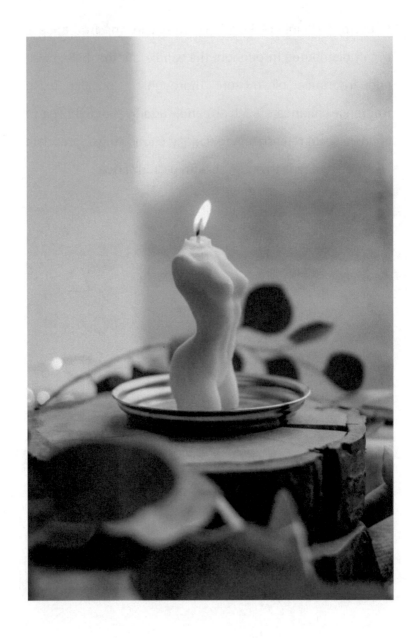

Conclusion: Incorporating fragrances into candles is a creative and enjoyable process that allows fragrance lovers and DIY enthusiasts to craft personalized scents. By following the techniques discussed in this subchapter, you can create candles that not only look beautiful but also fill your space with captivating aromas. Whether you are making candles for personal use or for an e-commerce business, these techniques will help you master the art of candle fragrance formulation.

Chapter 12: Fragrance Formulation for Bath and Body Products

Introduction to Bath and Body Products

Bath and body products are an essential part of our daily self-care routine. Whether it's a luxurious bubble bath, a moisturizing body lotion, or a fragrant soap, these products not only cleanse and nourish our skin but also provide a sensory experience that enhances our overall well-being.

In this subchapter, we will delve into the fascinating world of bath and body products and explore the various aspects of creating and using them. Whether you are a fragrance lover, a DIY enthusiast, or an e-commerce entrepreneur looking to expand your product line, this chapter is designed to provide you with a comprehensive introduction to this exciting field.

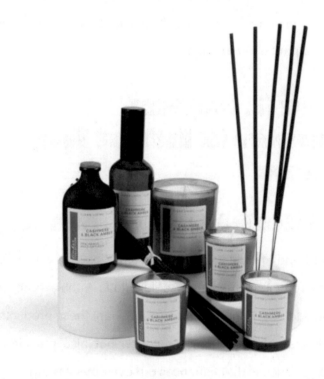

Beginners in the art of perfume making will find this subchapter particularly valuable as it touches upon the fundamentals of creating signature scents and fragrance layering techniques. Understanding how different fragrance notes interact with each other and how to blend them harmoniously is essential for anyone interested in making their own fragrances.

Additionally, we will explore the world of natural fragrances and the benefits of incorporating aromatherapy into your fragrance blends. Discover the healing properties of essential oils and learn how to create customized fragrance oils that cater to specific needs, such as relaxation, stress relief, or energy boost.

For those interested in replicating vintage perfumes, we will provide insights into the art of vintage perfume replication. Uncover the secrets of classic fragrances and recreate their olfactory magic with your own unique twist.

Furthermore, we will explore the world of solid perfume making, a convenient and portable alternative to traditional liquid perfumes. Learn how to create solid perfume balms that can be easily applied and carried with you throughout the day.

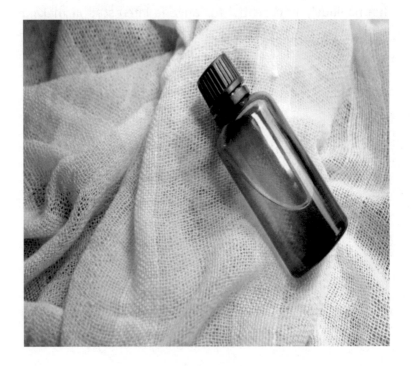

Lastly, we will touch upon the fascinating subject of fragrance formulation for bath and body products. Discover the art of creating scented candles, lotions, and soaps that not only smell divine but also provide nourishment and hydration to the skin. Explore different fragrance families and learn how to formulate balanced and long-lasting fragrances for your bath and body products.

Whether you are a hobbyist, a DIY enthusiast, or an aspiring entrepreneur, this subchapter will equip you with the knowledge and skills to embark on your journey of creating and enjoying bath and body products. So, dive in and explore the wonderful world of fragrance formulation for bath and body products!

Fragrance Selection for Different Products

When it comes to creating your own fragrances, selecting the right scent for each product is crucial. The aroma you choose can make or break the overall experience for your customers. In this subchapter, we will explore the art of fragrance selection for different products, ensuring that you create delightful scents that cater to a variety of needs and preferences.

How to make Fragrances: For those who are new to perfume making, understanding the process of fragrance selection is essential. We will guide you through the different fragrance families and teach you how to create harmonious blends that appeal to your own unique taste.

DIY Natural Fragrances: If you prefer working with natural ingredients, this section will provide you with insights on selecting essential oils and plant-based materials to create your own natural fragrances. We will discuss the benefits of using natural ingredients and provide tips on achieving the perfect balance between scents.

Perfume Making for Beginners: As a beginner, navigating the vast world of perfumery can be overwhelming. We will simplify the process by sharing our expert tips on selecting the right fragrance notes for your perfume. You will learn about top, middle, and base notes, and how to combine them to create a well-rounded fragrance.

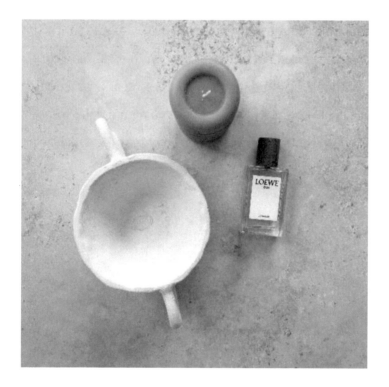

Aromatherapy Fragrance Blending: Aromatherapy is a powerful tool for relaxation and well-being. In this section, we will explore the art of blending fragrances specifically for aromatherapy purposes. You will discover the therapeutic properties of different essential oils and learn how to create blends that promote relaxation, focus, or upliftment.

Creating Signature Scents: Whether you are a perfume enthusiast or an entrepreneur looking to establish your own fragrance brand, creating a signature scent is essential. We will delve into the process of developing a unique fragrance that represents your personal style or brand identity, helping you stand out in a crowded market.

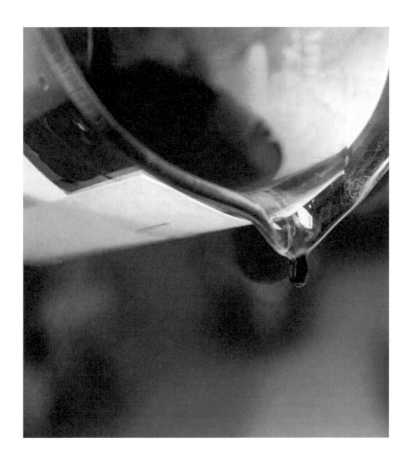

Vintage Perfume Replication: Vintage perfumes have a timeless appeal. In this section, we will explore the art of replicating vintage fragrances, allowing you to recreate beloved scents from the past. We will guide you through the process of researching and sourcing the necessary ingredients to bring these classic perfumes back to life.

Fragrance Layering Techniques: Layering fragrances is a popular technique used to create complex and unique scents. We will teach you how to layer different fragrances to achieve a harmonious blend that is both captivating and long-lasting.

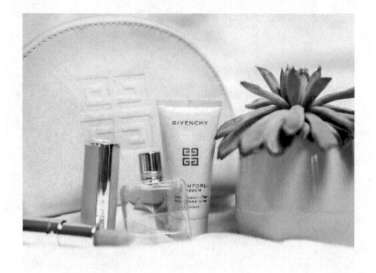

Solid Perfume Making: Solid perfumes offer a convenient and portable alternative to traditional liquid perfumes. In this section, we will guide you through the process of creating solid perfumes, including selecting the right fragrance notes and incorporating them into a solid base.

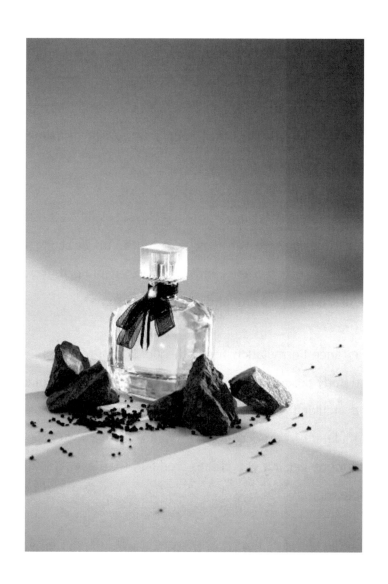

Customized Fragrance Oils: Fragrance oils are widely used in various products, including candles, soaps, and bath and body products. We will discuss the process of formulating customized fragrance oils to suit specific product requirements, ensuring that your creations have a unique and captivating scent.

Scented Candle Making: Fragrance plays a significant role in candle making. We will provide insights into selecting the right fragrance oils for candle making, ensuring that your candles emit a pleasant and long-lasting aroma.

Fragrance Formulation for Bath and Body Products: Bath and body products rely on fragrances to create a luxurious and indulgent experience. We will discuss the process of formulating fragrances for bath salts, shower gels, lotions, and more, helping you create products that leave a lasting impression.

By understanding the art of fragrance selection for different products, you will be able to create captivating scents that cater to the diverse needs and preferences of fragrance lovers, DIY enthusiasts, and e-commerce entrepreneurs. Embark on this fragrant journey and unlock the endless possibilities of perfume making.

Balancing Fragrance with Other Ingredients

In the world of perfume making, the fragrance itself is undoubtedly the star of the show. However, it is essential to understand that creating a well-rounded and harmonious scent requires more than just a beautiful fragrance. Balancing fragrance with other ingredients is crucial to achieve the desired outcome in your perfume creations.

When formulating a perfume, it is important to consider the different notes that make up the fragrance. These notes are categorized into top, middle, and base notes, each playing a unique role in the overall scent composition. While the fragrance oils provide the main aroma, other ingredients such as carrier oils, alcohol, and fixatives help enhance and stabilize the scent.

One key consideration when balancing fragrance with other ingredients is to ensure that the supporting components do not overpower or dilute the fragrance itself. The goal is to create a harmonious blend where each ingredient complements the fragrance without overshadowing it. This requires careful measurement and experimentation to find the perfect balance.

Carrier oils are commonly used in perfume making to dilute the fragrance oils and to provide a medium for the scent to linger on the skin. Different carrier oils have varying levels of scent absorption, so it is important to choose one that does not alter the fragrance but rather enhances its longevity.

Alcohol is another ingredient often used in perfumes to help disperse the fragrance and provide a quick-drying effect. However, it is crucial to strike the right balance as too much alcohol can evaporate the fragrance too quickly, while too little can make the scent heavy and overpowering.

Fixatives are substances that help stabilize the fragrance and slow down its evaporation. They are essential in ensuring that the scent lingers on the skin for a longer period. Common fixatives include musk, ambergris, and benzoin.

In addition to these supporting ingredients, understanding the art of blending is crucial in achieving a well-balanced fragrance. Experimenting with different combinations of notes, layering techniques, and vintage perfume replication can help create unique and personalized scents.

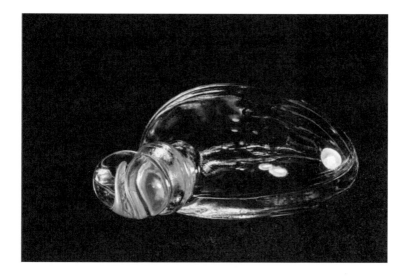

Whether you are a fragrance lover, DIY enthusiast, or e-commerce entrepreneur, mastering the art of balancing fragrance with other ingredients is essential in perfume making. It allows you to create signature scents, replicate vintage perfumes, and formulate fragrances for various products such as candles and bath and body products.

By understanding the role of carrier oils, alcohol, fixatives, and the art of blending, you can take your perfume making skills to the next level. With practice and experimentation, you will be able to create beautiful and well-balanced fragrances that leave a lasting impression.

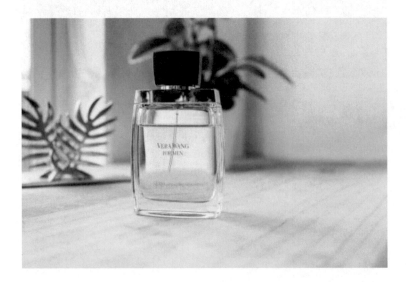

Chapter 13: Packaging and Marketing Your Perfume Creations

Choosing the Right Packaging Materials

When it comes to packaging your homemade fragrances, it's important to select the right materials that not only protect your products but also enhance their appeal. The packaging you choose plays a crucial role in attracting customers, keeping your creations safe, and maintaining their quality. In this subchapter, we will explore the different types of packaging materials available and help you make informed decisions tailored to your specific needs.

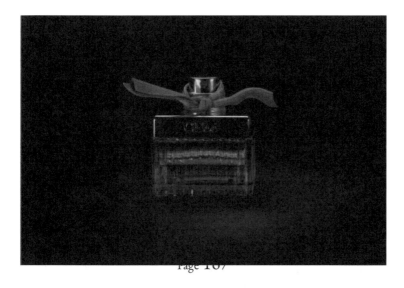

For fragrances, it is recommended to opt for packaging materials that are both aesthetically pleasing and functional. Glass bottles are a popular choice due to their elegance and ability to preserve the fragrance's integrity. Amber or dark-colored glass bottles are particularly beneficial as they provide UV protection, preventing light from deteriorating the scent over time. Additionally, glass bottles are easy to clean and refill, making them a sustainable option.

For those interested in DIY natural fragrances, consider using eco-friendly packaging materials. Bamboo or wooden containers not only add a touch of natural beauty but also align with the values of sustainability and environmental consciousness. These materials are biodegradable and can be easily repurposed or recycled, minimizing your ecological footprint.

If you are an e-commerce business, it is crucial to prioritize packaging materials that are lightweight, durable, and offer protection during shipping. Air-tight and leak-proof containers are essential to prevent any spillage or damage to your products during transit. Look for packaging options that include secure closures, such as screw caps or dropper assemblies, to ensure the perfume remains intact throughout its journey.

For those interested in creating signature scents, consider using customizable packaging materials. Some manufacturers offer the option to design unique labels, allowing you to add a personal touch to your products. This is especially beneficial for those in niche markets, as it helps create brand recognition and sets your fragrances apart from competitors.

Lastly, consider the cost-effectiveness of your packaging materials. As a beginner, it is important to balance quality and affordability. Evaluate different options and compare prices to find the best fit for your budget without compromising on the overall quality and aesthetic appeal.

By choosing the right packaging materials, you can enhance the overall experience for your customers and ensure that your fragrances are well-protected and presented. Whether you're creating signature scents, DIY natural fragrances, or exploring the world of vintage perfume replication, selecting the appropriate packaging materials is a crucial step in your perfume-making journey.

Labeling and Branding Your Perfume Products

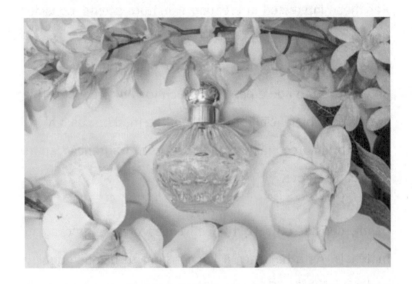

When it comes to selling perfume products, labeling and branding play a vital role in attracting customers and creating a strong identity for your brand. In this subchapter, we will explore the essential aspects of labeling and branding your perfume products, providing you with valuable insights and tips to make your fragrances stand out in a competitive market.

Labeling is not just about adding a name and ingredients list to your perfume bottles; it is an opportunity to showcase your brand's personality and create a visual representation of your product. Start by designing a unique and eye-catching logo that reflects the essence of your brand. This logo will be the face of your perfume line, so ensure it is memorable and easily recognizable.

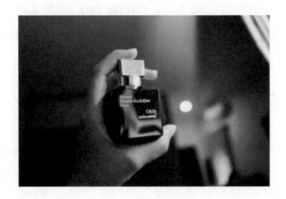

Once you have a logo, incorporate it into your labels, which should be professionally printed for a polished and high-quality look. Consider using high-quality materials for your labels, such as textured paper or glossy finishes, to add a touch of luxury to your packaging.

In addition to your logo, include essential information on your labels, such as the name of the perfume, the volume or size of the product, the list of ingredients (in compliance with regulatory requirements), and your brand's contact information. This information not only ensures compliance with labeling regulations but also helps customers make informed choices.

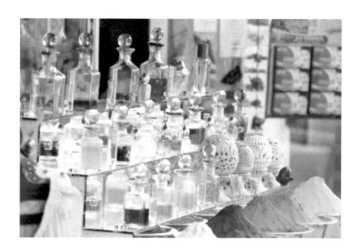

When it comes to branding, consistency is key. Ensure that your branding elements, such as your logo, color palette, and font choices, are consistent across all your marketing materials, including

your website, social media profiles, and product packaging. This consistency creates a cohesive and recognizable brand identity that customers can trust.

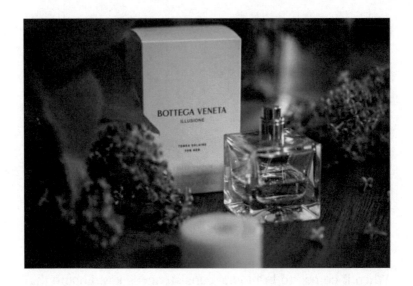

Consider creating a unique and compelling brand story to accompany your perfume products. Share the inspiration behind your fragrances, the sourcing of your ingredients, or the craftsmanship involved in the creation process. This story will engage customers on an emotional level and differentiate your brand from others in the market.

Lastly, remember to tailor your labeling and branding to your target audience. Fragrance lovers, DIY enthusiasts, and e-commerce customers all have different preferences and expectations. Research your target audience's tastes and preferences to create labels and branding elements that resonate with them.

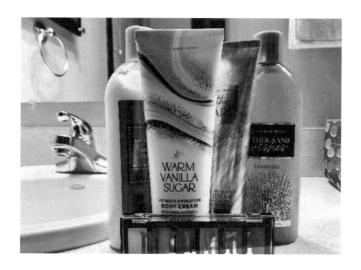

By carefully designing labels and branding your perfume products, you can create a strong brand identity and attract customers in the fragrance market. So, take the time to invest in professional labeling and branding that aligns with your brand's values and appeals to your target audience.

Strategies for Selling Your Perfumes Online and Offline

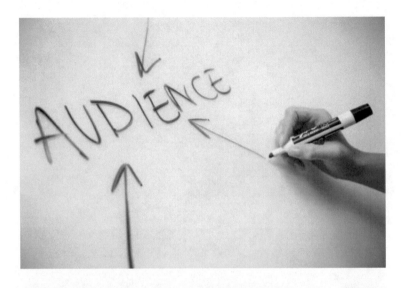

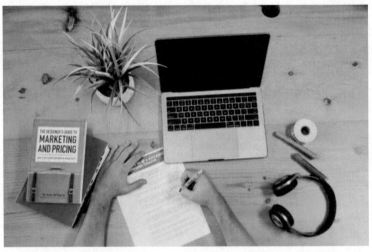

In the digital age, selling your perfumes online and offline requires a combination of effective marketing strategies and a solid understanding of your target audience. Whether you are a fragrance lover, DIY enthusiast, or e-commerce entrepreneur, the following strategies will help you successfully sell your perfumes and connect with your customers.

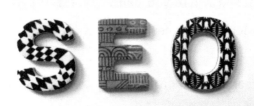

Online Strategies: 1. Build an Engaging Website: Create a user-friendly website that showcases your perfumes and provides detailed descriptions, ingredients, and testimonials. Incorporate high-quality product images and an easy-to-use checkout process. 2. Utilize Social Media: Leverage social media platforms such as Instagram, Facebook, and Pinterest to showcase your perfumes visually. Share engaging content, including tutorials, behind- the-scenes glimpses, and customer reviews. Engage with your audience through comments and direct messages. 3. Offer Personalized Fragrance Consultations: Provide online consultations where you can recommend perfumes based on individual preferences and personalities.

This personalized approach helps customers feel connected and confident in their purchase decisions. 4.

Collaborate with Influencers: Partner with fragrance influencers or bloggers to promote your perfumes. Offer them samples to review and share their experiences with their followers. This can significantly boost your online visibility and credibility.

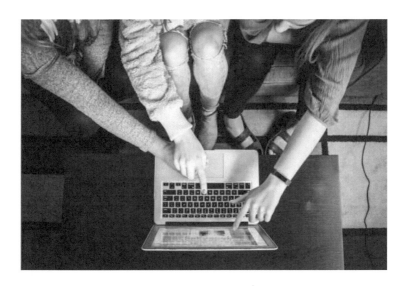

Offline Strategies: 1. Participate in Trade Shows and Exhibitions: Showcase your perfumes at local trade shows or fragrance exhibitions. This allows you to engage directly with potential customers, receive feedback, and build brand recognition. 2. Collaborate with Local Retailers: Approach local boutiques, spas, or beauty salons to stock your perfumes. Offer them attractive wholesale pricing and display materials to promote your brand effectively. 3. Organize Perfume-Making Workshops: Host workshops where participants can learn the art of perfume-making. This not only generates direct revenue but also establishes you as an expert in the field and promotes your products.

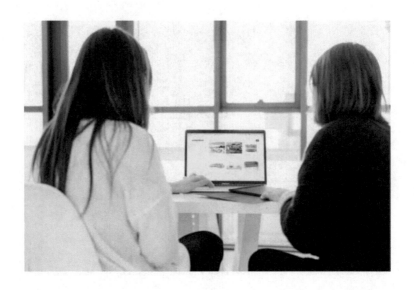

4. Offer Samples and Trial Sizes: Provide small sample sizes or trial kits that allow customers to experience your perfumes before committing to a full-size purchase. This strategy encourages them to try new scents and increases the likelihood of repeat sales. 5. Create Gift Sets and Limited Editions: Design exclusive gift sets or limited-edition collections that attract attention and create a sense of urgency. This scarcity mindset can drive sales and foster customer loyalty.

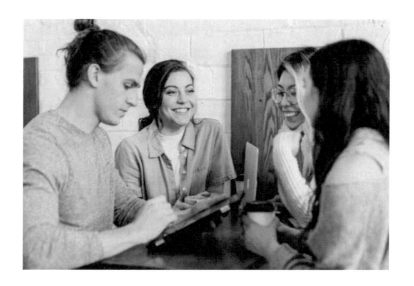

By implementing these strategies, you can effectively sell your perfumes both online and offline. Remember to continuously analyze customer feedback, adapt your marketing approach, and stay updated with industry trends to achieve long-term success in the competitive fragrance market.

Chapter 14: Troubleshooting and Tips for Perfume Making

Common Perfume Making Problems and Solutions

Perfume making is an art that combines creativity and scientific precision. It offers fragrance lovers, DIY enthusiasts, and e-commerce entrepreneurs the opportunity to create unique scents that reflect their personality or cater to a specific market. However, like any creative endeavor, perfume making can present its fair share of challenges. In this subchapter, we will explore some common perfume making problems and provide practical solutions to help you overcome them.

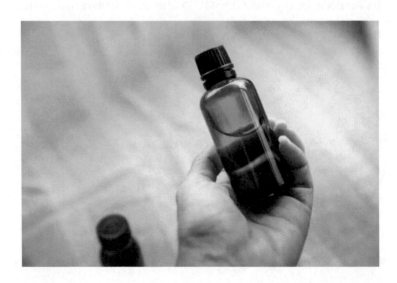

One frequent issue encountered by beginners is the lack of longevity in their fragrances. You may find that your perfume fades quickly or doesn't last as long as commercial perfumes. The solution lies in understanding the fragrance pyramid and adjusting the concentration of your fragrance oils accordingly. Top notes, which provide the initial burst of scent, are usually volatile and evaporate quickly. By increasing the concentration of middle and base notes, which have a longer staying power, you can enhance the longevity of your perfume.

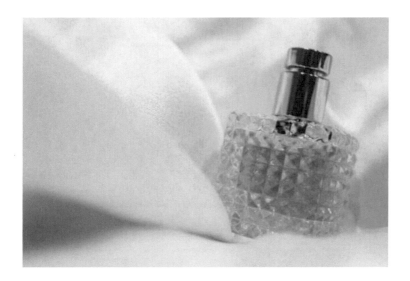

Another common problem is the lack of balance in a perfume's composition. Sometimes, certain ingredients can overpower the scent, making it unappealing or unbalanced. To address this, experiment with different ingredient ratios and consider the interplay of fragrances within the fragrance families. A good rule of thumb is to start with a smaller quantity of strong or overpowering ingredients and gradually increase as needed.

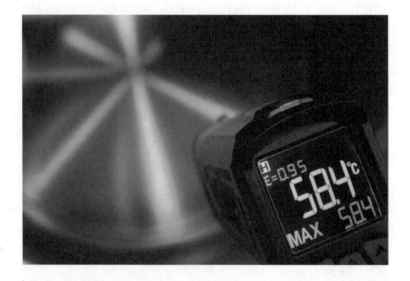

Storage and preservation are also crucial aspects of perfume making. Improper storage can lead to oxidation, discoloration, and loss of fragrance potency. To prevent this, store your perfumes in dark, airtight bottles away from direct sunlight and extreme temperatures. Additionally, adding a few drops of Vitamin E oil to your perfume can act as a natural preservative, prolonging its shelf life.

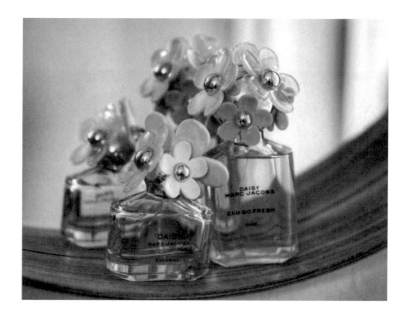

One last challenge to address is the difficulty in sourcing unique or rare fragrance oils. While commercial suppliers offer a wide range of options, they may not always carry the exact ingredients you desire. In such cases, consider reaching out to boutique suppliers or exploring online communities dedicated to perfume making. Networking with fellow fragrance enthusiasts can provide valuable insights and recommendations for sourcing hard-to-find fragrance oils.

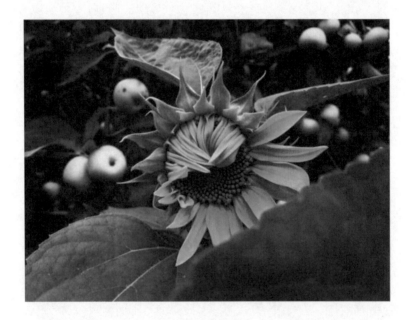

Perfume making is a journey of trial and error, but with these solutions, you can overcome common challenges and create exceptional fragrances. By understanding the science behind perfume composition, experimenting with ingredient ratios, and ensuring proper storage, you will be well on your way to mastering the art of perfume making. Whether you are a fragrance lover, a DIY enthusiast, or an aspiring e-commerce entrepreneur, this subchapter will equip you with the knowledge and tools to create fragrances that captivate the senses and leave a lasting impression.

Tips for Enhancing Longevity and Projection of Scents

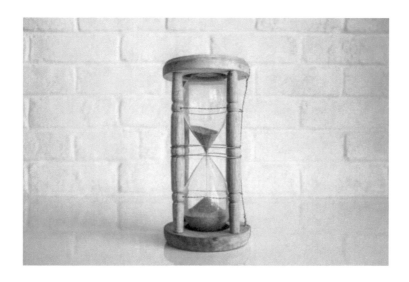

When it comes to creating your own perfumes, achieving a long-lasting scent with good projection is key. After all, what's the point of crafting a beautiful fragrance if it doesn't last or project well? In this subchapter, we will explore some essential tips and techniques to help you enhance the longevity and projection of your scents, empowering you to create captivating fragrances that leave a lasting impression. 1. Concentration is Key: Choosing the right concentration of fragrance oils is crucial to ensure longevity and projection. Higher concentrations, such as eau de parfum (EDP) or perfume oils, tend to have a longer-lasting effect. Experiment with different concentrations to find your desired balance.

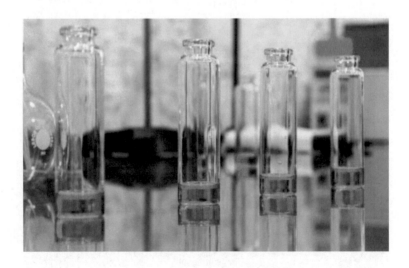

2. Base Notes: Incorporating strong base notes into your perfume formula can significantly enhance longevity.

Base notes like vanilla, amber, or musk have a long-lasting effect and help anchor the scent throughout the day. Experiment with different base notes to find the perfect combination for your fragrance. 3. Fixatives: Including fixatives in your perfume formulation helps to retain the fragrance on the skin for a longer duration. Common fixatives include benzoin, orris root, and tonka bean. These fixatives not only prolong the scent but also add depth and complexity to your fragrance. 4. Layering Technique: Layering scents is a great way to enhance projection. Start by applying a matching scented body lotion or oil before spritzing your perfume. The moisturized skin holds the fragrance better, allowing it to project more effectively throughout the day. 5.

Application Points: Knowing where and how to apply your perfume can also impact its longevity and projection.

Apply your fragrance to pulse points such as the wrists, neck, behind the ears, and inside the elbows. These areas generate heat, which helps to release the fragrance gradually. 6. Storage: Proper storage of your perfumes is essential to maintain their quality. Keep your fragrances away from direct sunlight and store them in cool, dark places. Exposure to heat and light can degrade the scent molecules, reducing their longevity. 7. Quality Ingredients: Using high-quality fragrance oils and ingredients is crucial for achieving a long-lasting scent. Invest in good quality essential oils, aroma chemicals, and carrier oils to ensure the longevity and projection of your fragrances.

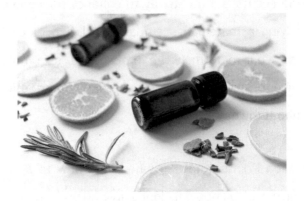

By following these tips and techniques, you can enhance the longevity and projection of your homemade perfumes. Remember, fragrance-making is an art, and experimentation is key to finding the perfect balance that suits your preferences. With practice and the right techniques, you can create captivating scents that leave a lasting impression on yourself and others.

Storing and Preserving Perfume Formulas

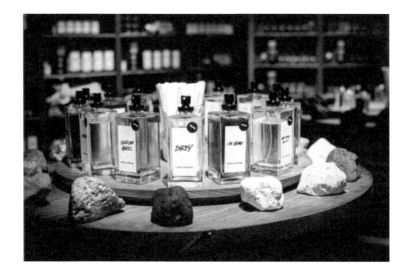

When it comes to perfume making, one of the most important aspects to consider is the proper storage and preservation of your precious fragrance formulas. Whether you are a fragrance lover, a DIY enthusiast, or an e-commerce entrepreneur, understanding the best practices for storing and preserving perfume formulas is essential for maintaining the quality and longevity of your creations.

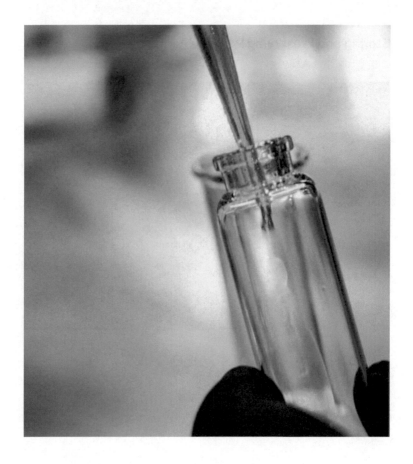

First and foremost, it is crucial to store your perfume formulas in a cool, dark, and dry place. Heat, light, and humidity can all have a detrimental effect on the stability and composition of your fragrances. Therefore, it is recommended to store your perfume formulas in airtight containers, preferably made of glass or aluminum, which can provide maximum protection from external factors.

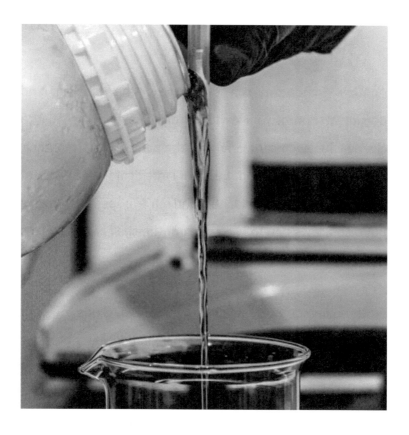

Additionally, it is vital to keep your perfume formulas away from any strong odors or chemicals. Perfumes are highly sensitive to external influences, and exposure to strong scents or chemicals can alter the fragrance profile or even cause it to become rancid. Therefore, it is advisable to store your perfume formulas separately, in a dedicated space away from other substances.

Another important consideration is the labeling and documentation of your perfume formulas. It is essential to clearly label each container with the name of the fragrance, the date of creation, and the list of ingredients used. This not only helps you to easily identify and retrieve specific formulas but also allows you to keep track of the shelf life and usage of each perfume.

Furthermore, it is beneficial to create backups of your perfume formulas. Accidents happen, and losing a precious formula can be devastating. By keeping multiple copies of your formulas, either in digital or physical form, you can ensure that you always have a backup in case of any unforeseen circumstances.

Lastly, it is advisable to regularly check the condition and quality of your stored perfume formulas. Over time, even with proper storage, fragrances may undergo changes due to aging or exposure to air. By periodically assessing the scent, color, and overall quality of your stored perfumes, you can identify any potential issues and take necessary steps to rectify them.

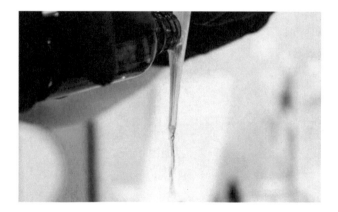

In conclusion, storing and preserving perfume formulas is a crucial aspect of perfume making. By following these guidelines and best practices, fragrance lovers, DIY enthusiasts, and e-commerce entrepreneurs can ensure the longevity and quality of their creations, allowing them to enjoy and share their unique fragrances for years to come.

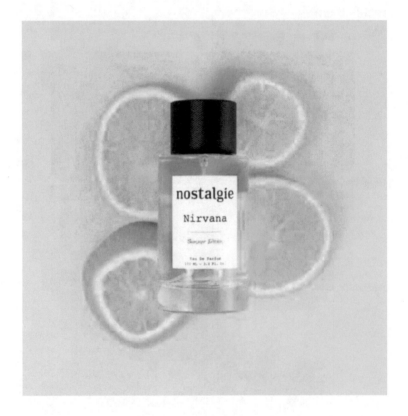

Chapter 15: Advanced Perfume Making Techniques (Optional)

Exploring Advanced Blending Techniques

In the exciting world of perfume making, mastering the art of blending is key to creating unique and captivating fragrances. While beginners may start with simple scent combinations, advanced blending techniques allow fragrance enthusiasts to push the boundaries of creativity and unleash their olfactory imagination. In this subchapter, we will delve into the realm of advanced blending techniques, uncovering the secrets behind creating complex and harmonious aromas.

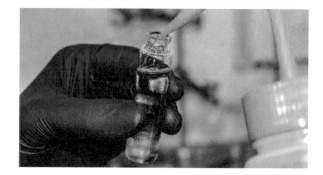

One technique that experienced perfumers often employ is called layering. This method involves building a fragrance by adding multiple layers of different scents, allowing each layer to fully develop before adding the next. Layering allows for the creation of intricate perfumes with a rich and multi-dimensional character. Fragrance lovers will learn how to carefully select and combine various top, middle, and base notes to achieve a harmonious blend that evolves over time.

Another advanced blending technique that will be explored is accords. Accords are specific combinations of scents that create a unique aroma or impression. By understanding the different families of fragrances and their key characteristics, DIY perfume makers can experiment with blending various accords to achieve a desired scent profile. From floral and citrus accords to woody and oriental accords, the possibilities are endless.

Furthermore, this subchapter will introduce fragrance lovers to the concept of modifying existing fragrances. By understanding the components of a perfume and how they interact, individuals can personalize and enhance commercially available scents. Whether it's adjusting the longevity, adding a touch of freshness, or introducing a new note, these advanced blending techniques provide the opportunity to create a signature fragrance that truly reflects one's individual style.

For those interested in the e-commerce aspect of perfume making, this subchapter will also touch upon the importance of branding and marketing. The niche of "How to make Fragrances" offers a vast array of possibilities for entrepreneurs to establish their own unique brand and stand out in a competitive market. Understanding the target audience, packaging, and effective storytelling techniques will be explored to help fragrance enthusiasts succeed in the e-commerce space.

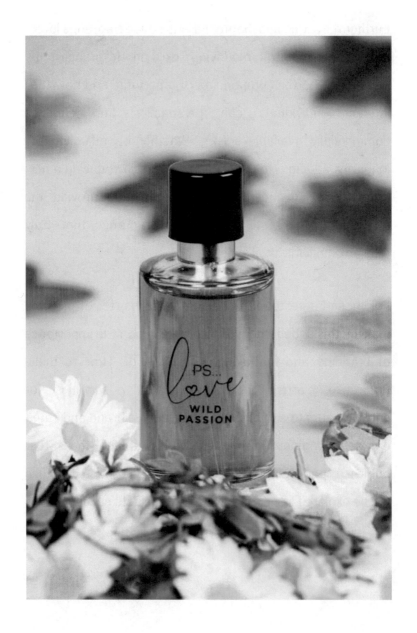

In conclusion, exploring advanced blending techniques opens up a world of possibilities for fragrance lovers, DIY enthusiasts, and those interested in the e-commerce niche of perfume making. By mastering layering, accords, and modification, individuals can create captivating and personalized fragrances that will leave a lasting impression. So, let your creativity run wild and embark on a scented journey like no other with the knowledge gained from this subchapter.

Incorporating Rare and Exotic Ingredients

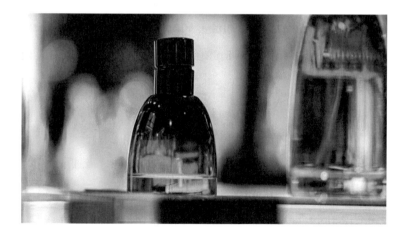

One of the most exciting aspects of perfume making is the ability to experiment with rare and exotic ingredients. These unique elements can add depth, complexity, and intrigue to your fragrances, elevating them to a whole new level. In this subchapter, we will explore the world of rare and exotic ingredients and discuss how to incorporate them into your perfume creations.

When it comes to rare and exotic ingredients, the possibilities are endless. From precious flowers like jasmine and rose to rare spices like cardamom and saffron, there is no shortage of options to choose from. These ingredients are often sourced from remote regions around the world, making them not only unique but also imbued with a sense of adventure and discovery.

To incorporate rare and exotic ingredients into your perfumes, it is essential to start by understanding their characteristics and olfactory profiles. Each ingredient has its own distinct scent, with some being more dominant and others playing supporting roles. By studying and familiarizing yourself with these scents, you can begin to envision how they will interact with other components in your fragrance.

When working with rare and exotic ingredients, it is crucial to use them sparingly. Due to their scarcity and high cost, these ingredients are often more valuable than their more common counterparts. Using them in small quantities will not only help you stretch your supply but also ensure that their unique qualities are not overwhelmed by other elements in your perfume.

Furthermore, it is essential to consider the balance and harmony of your fragrance composition. Rare and exotic ingredients can be potent, so it is crucial to strike the right balance between them and other components. Experimentation and testing are key in finding the perfect blend that showcases the unique qualities of these ingredients without overpowering the overall composition.

For fragrance lovers, DIY enthusiasts, and e-commerce entrepreneurs, incorporating rare and exotic ingredients into your perfume creations can provide a competitive edge in the market. Consumers are always on the lookout for unique and intriguing scents that set them apart from the crowd. By utilizing these rare and exotic ingredients, you can create fragrances that are truly one-of-a-kind, captivating the senses and leaving a lasting impression.

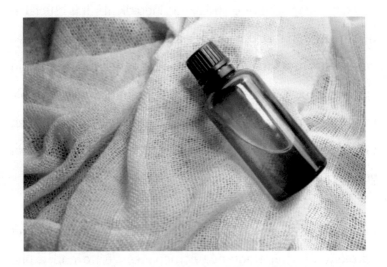

In conclusion, incorporating rare and exotic ingredients into your perfume creations is an exciting and rewarding endeavor. By understanding the characteristics of these ingredients, using them sparingly, and finding the right balance, you can create fragrances that are truly exceptional. Whether you are a fragrance lover, a DIY enthusiast, or an e-commerce entrepreneur, exploring the world of rare and exotic ingredients will open up a new world of possibilities in your perfume making journey.

Pushing Boundaries and Creating Unique Fragrance Experiences

In the world of fragrance, there is an endless array of scents waiting to be discovered and created. For fragrance lovers, DIY enthusiasts, and e-commerce entrepreneurs, the art of making fragrances offers a unique opportunity to explore and push boundaries in the realm of scent.

Creating your own fragrance is a journey that allows you to unleash your creativity and express your unique personality. It's not just about following a set of instructions; it's about experimenting,

exploring different combinations, and finding the perfect blend that resonates with your senses. With the right guidance and a step-by-step approach, anyone can learn the art of perfume making.

This subchapter delves into the exciting realm of pushing boundaries and creating unique fragrance experiences. It explores the techniques and approaches that fragrance enthusiasts can use to create one-of-a-kind scents that stand out from the crowd.

One way to push boundaries is by experimenting with unconventional ingredients and combinations. By stepping away from the traditional fragrance notes and exploring unusual aromas, you can create fragrances that are unexpected and captivating. This subchapter will guide you through the process of sourcing and incorporating unique ingredients, opening up a world of possibilities for your fragrance creations.

Additionally, it will delve into the concept of layering scents to create complex and multi-dimensional fragrances. By understanding the various fragrance families and their compatibility, you can create captivating combinations that evolve over time, offering a truly unique olfactory experience.

For those in the e-commerce niche, this subchapter will provide insights on how to market and sell your unique fragrances. It will explore strategies for creating compelling product descriptions, captivating visuals, and engaging storytelling that will resonate with your target audience.

Whether you are a fragrance lover, a DIY enthusiast, or an e-commerce entrepreneur, this subchapter will empower you to take your fragrance creations to the next level. By pushing boundaries and exploring new frontiers in scent, you can create truly unique fragrance experiences that leave a lasting impression on those who encounter them. So dive in, let your creativity flow, and embark on a fragrant journey like no other.

Conclusion: Embrace Your Fragrance Journey

Congratulations! You have completed your fragrance journey and are now equipped with the knowledge and skills to create your own unique scents. Throughout this book, we have delved into the fascinating world of perfume making, providing you with a step-by-step guide that demystifies the process and encourages your creativity to flourish. Now, it's time for you to embrace your fragrance journey and explore the endless possibilities that await you.

For fragrance lovers, this book has opened up a whole new avenue of enjoyment. You no longer need to rely solely on commercial perfumes; instead, you can create your own signature scent that perfectly captures your personality and style. Imagine the joy of wearing a fragrance that is truly one- of-a-kind, crafted with love and care. The sense of accomplishment and satisfaction that comes with creating your own perfume is unparalleled.

DIY enthusiasts will find this book to be an invaluable resource. Perfume making is a rewarding and fulfilling hobby that allows you to express your creativity and experiment with different ingredients and combinations. You can now impress your friends and family with your homemade fragrances, and even turn your passion into a small business. The possibilities for DIY perfume making are endless, and the journey is as exciting as the end result.

E-commerce entrepreneurs will discover new opportunities in the fragrance industry. With the knowledge gained from this book, you can develop your own line of perfumes, tapping into the growing demand for niche and artisanal fragrances. Whether you choose to create your own brand or collaborate with established perfumers, the insights and techniques shared in this book will give you a competitive edge in the market.

In conclusion, "Perfume Making for Beginners: A Step-by-Step Guide" has taken you on an immersive journey into the world of fragrance creation. It has empowered you to explore your creativity, experiment with different scents, and develop your own unique blends. Embrace this

newfound knowledge and let your fragrance journey continue to evolve. Whether you are a fragrance lover, a DIY enthusiast, or an e-commerce entrepreneur, the art of perfume making offers endless possibilities. So, seize the opportunity, trust your nose, and embark on an exciting fragrance adventure that is truly yours. Happy perfume making!

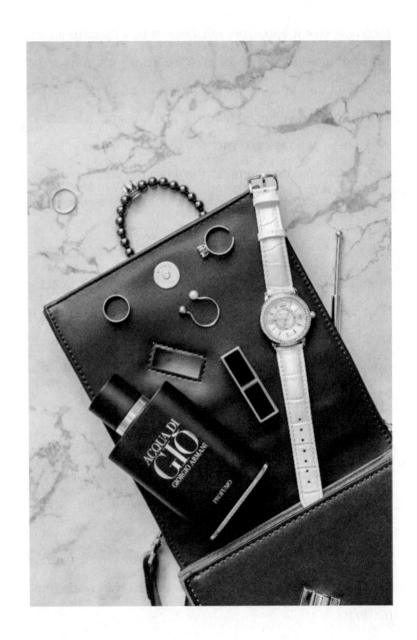

Made in the USA
Columbia, SC
21 September 2024

42737861R00115